MW00534146

Move Like a Champion®

The Power of Understanding How Your Body Works

Diane Jarmolow and **Kasia Kozak**

with **Brandee Selck**

The information presented in this book is intended for educational purposes only and is not a substitute for medical advice or treatment by a health care professional. If you feel any discomfort or pain while doing an exercise, stop and consult your doctor or other qualified professional.

Copyright 2011 by Move Like a Champion Inc. All rights reserved.

No part of this book may be reproduced in any form or by any electronic or mechanical means (including information storage and retrieval systems) without written permission by the publisher. Move Like a Champion Inc. will prosecute any individual or company, within the United States or any other country, who reproduces any or all of this text without the express written permission of its publisher. Move Like a Champion Inc. offers a reward of $1000 for information leading to the prosecution of copyright infringement upon its property.

All photos copyright by Jonathan Marion. Photos may not be reproduced in any form without express written permission from the photographer.

Move Like a Champion® is a registered trademark of Move Like a Champion Inc. *Teach Like a Pro*® is a registered trademark of Ballroom Dance Teachers College. All other trademarks are acknowledged as property of their owners.

Cover design by Brion Sausser (bookcreatives.com), inspired by Dani Palmer's original design
Dancers featured on cover are Gherman Mustuc and Iveta Lukosiute, 2008-2010 World Professional 10 Dance Champions

Book design by Brandee Selck

Photography by Jonathan Marion

Corrections: We are committed to updating and improving our product so that you can count on its accuracy. If you find an error, please email movelikeachampion@gmail.com Please be sure to include the exercise and page numbers in your email.

ISBN 978-0-615-45547-1

"The same amount of time is needed to be an artist in the control of the body as an artist in physics, music, art, or anything else." - Moshe Feldenkrais

"If you know what you are doing, you can do what you want." - Moshe Feldenkrais

"Our bodies communicate to us clearly and specifically, if we are willing to listen." - Shakti Gawain

"Our own physical body possesses a wisdom which we who inhabit the body lack - we give it orders which make no sense." - Henry Miller

"You can't tell a person what to do, because the thing you have to do is a sensation." - F. M. Alexander

"If it feels right on the inside, it will be right on the outside." - Luigi

"The real message of the Dance opens up the vistas of life to all who have the urge to express beauty with no other instrument than their own bodies, with no apparatus and no dependence on anything other than space." - Ruth St. Denis

Table of Contents

Acknowledgements

Over the course of our careers, a variety of people have contributed to our understanding of ballroom dance and the way the human body moves. However, there are a few who have particularly influenced our thinking and been an inspiration for the creation of *Move Like a Champion*. We gratefully acknowledge the invaluable resource the following have been for the exercises in this book:

Dr. Moshe Feldenkrais and the *Feldenkrais Method*®, movement education that uses awareness to recognize our habits and organic learning to improve movement and overall functioning.

Ruthy Alon and the Bones for Life® program, movement education that stimulates efficient weight-bearing posture to maintain healthy bones, improve movement and increase vitality.

Eric Franklin and the Franklin-Method, movement education for dancers emphasizing dynamic alignment, experiential anatomy and the use of imagery for maximum efficiency.

Luigi (Louis Facciuto), jazz dance innovator who promotes the importance of dancers using their bodies properly and taking time to *feel* what they are doing.

Dr. Eric Cobb and Z Health® Performance Solutions, a system of joint-specific exercises that improves coordination, agility, control and overall performance.

We would also like to personally thank the following individuals for their support: Lin Maxwell, Jennifer Bury, David Weise, Tom Slater, Theresa Nesbitt and Marcin Tomaszewski (our wonderful model).

Preface

We all marvel at the amazing grace, power, precision and effortlessness exuded by champion dancers. Many of us may think this level of mastery is not possible for us. While not everyone becomes a champion, the possibilities for improvement in our dancing are truly limitless—we just need the right tools and approach to learning.

Usually when dancers practice, they watch and imitate good dancers, use mirrors to see how they look, and try to apply their teachers' corrections. While useful to our learning, we will never achieve all that we are capable of through these methods alone. To realize our full potential we must use our sensitivity and intelligence to investigate *how* we move. *Move Like a Champion®* explores the use of our bones and joints, and the relationships between different parts of ourselves. It also includes slowing down when learning in order to sense ourselves, refine our movement, and eliminate extraneous efforts. This skillful use of attention has powerful, positive impact on our dancing, giving us the kinesthetic clarity to execute movements and technique just as we intend.

Until now ballroom dance training has not had the tools or language to teach how the body moves or develop internal awareness. *Move Like a Champion®* fills this gap, teaching these fundamental dance principles in a clear and accessible way. This training provides concrete understanding of human movement, resulting in greater flexibility, strength, balance and elegance—the qualities of champion dancers.

Diane Jarmolow has been dancing since 1978. She remembers feeling that there was a mystery about dance that made it difficult to learn. In 2002, she began studying Iyengar yoga, the yoga of body alignment. It was through this training that she learned how essential understanding how the body works is in creating good alignment and executing movements in the way you intend. As Diane started using the principles of yoga in her own dancing and teaching, she felt the mystery beginning to unravel. It then became her desire to codify this invaluable information into a fun and effective system for ballroom dancers.

Kasia Kozak has been dancing competitively since she was nine years old. She has always searched for ways to achieve perfection in dance technique and the physical capability to accomplish the movements required. Unlike many champions who limit their training to dance, Kasia has studied yoga, Pilates, Gyrotonics®, Z Health and Body

Mapping©. Her belief is that only with a comprehensive understanding of body movement can dance excellence truly be attained. Too often teachers refer students to outside sources to gain flexibility and strength because they themselves do not have the knowledge in these important areas. The *Move Like a Champion*® program gives teachers a fuller understanding of the body functions. They can use this knowledge to analyze and solve individual students' problems, allowing them to move forward with ease.

Brandee Selck began learning about movement via the *Feldenkrais Method*® in 1994, and started ballroom dancing a few years later. As a teacher, she found that many students had very little awareness of themselves and their movement —something which limited their ability to learn to dance. Wanting better tools with which to speed students' growth led her to become a *Guild Certified Feldenkrais Practitioner*cm. Brandee has contributed her knowledge of the body, movement and organic learning to the development of *Move Like a Champion*®, as well as her writing skills to document it in book form.

Introduction to Move Like a Champion

Accessible to All Dancers

Move Like a Champion® is a revolutionary training (and optional DVIDA® professional certification) that takes the mystery out of high-level dancing by distilling the techniques of ballroom champions. It is specifically designed for ballroom and Latin dancers (both students and teachers) who want to better understand how the body works to produce beautiful and efficient movement. The training teaches principles of dynamic alignment and functional movement through exercises and experiential anatomy. The comprehensive set of exercises increases awareness, develops all areas of the body, and can be applied to a wide range of dance styles and skill levels. The training also provides a standardized language with which to communicate these principles to dance partners and students. *Move Like a Champion*® is accessible to and beneficial for all dancers—from beginning student to champion dancer.

Benefits for Dance Students

If you are a brand new beginner taking dance lessons for fun and exercise, *Move Like a Champion*® will give you a tremendous boost. Not only will you more fully enjoy your dancing by being able to move easily and comfortably, but you will look and feel like a more experienced dancer. You will find that partners are eager to dance with you and fellow students notice how good your dancing has become.

If you are a student who performs, competes and/or takes medal tests, you need to learn everything you can to dance at a higher level. The foundational principles and exercises in *Move Like a Champion*® will help you achieve your goals. The exercises are great for warming up, fine tuning your technique, and correcting problem areas when they arise.

Benefits for Amateur and Professional Competitors

If you are a high level amateur or professional competitor, the information you attain in *Move Like a Champion*® will transform your dancing. The clarity you will gain about how and where movement is initiated will result in smoother, more efficient performance on the dance floor. Also, you will be able to produce the results your coaches are looking for by becoming more in tune with your body.

Benefits for Dance Teachers

If you are a dance teacher, *Move Like a Champion®* will raise the level of your teaching, improve your own dancing, and give you a competitive edge. You also have the ability to get DVIDA® certified (see next section)—an additional professional qualification with which to attract and retain students.

The *Move Like a Champion®* exercises integrate smoothly into lessons, and the results are immediately evident—your students will be dancing better than ever before! Based on what you observe during private lessons or a group class, simply introduce the appropriate exercises. For example, if you notice students' heads are drifting forward, you can remind them to use *Knuckle Biter!*, an exercise that activates the neck muscles to bring their heads into proper alignment. Or if you see students' dancing Tango with their pelvis tilted too far forward or back, simply call out *Don't Get Tipsy*, an exercise that brings the pelvis into a neutral alignment. The more you use this language in your own teaching and at your studio, the more progress and improvement you will see in your students.

Certification for Teachers

Why Get Certified?

To really learn a body of knowledge, we must make it a priority, take time to study, and be accountable to someone outside of ourselves. Becoming *Move Like a Champion®* DVIDA® certified demonstrates your dedication to professional excellence. It also provides you with the knowledge, skills and confidence to teach like a champion!

How Do I Get Certified?

After completing the training, you are eligible to take the certification exam. Preparation for the exam consists of learning all of the exercises and being able to teach them from memory. This is an easy task to accomplish—simply memorize a few exercises per day and start teaching them to your students. Within a few months you will be very comfortable teaching all the exercises.

The actual exam will be administered by Kasia Kozak or Diane Jarmolow (the *Move Like a Champion®* examiners). You will bring a student to whom you have *not* taught the exercises. The examiner will randomly choose 10 exercises, which you will then teach to your student. In addition, you will be examined on the names of the bones and joints covered in this book. After passing the exam, you will receive a certificate from ProDVIDA acknowledging your achievement. You can then advertise this prestigious certification along with your other professional accomplishments.

For More Information

For more information about *Move Like a Champion*® trainings or certification, please visit our website MoveLikeAChampion.com or email us at movelikeachampion@gmail.com.

How to Use This Book

Content and Organization

This book corresponds with the *Move Like a Champion*® Level 1 Training: How the Body Moves. It is designed to be compact and user friendly. Chapter 1 provides an orientation to the fundamental principles and terminology of *Move Like a Champion*®. The remaining chapters are arranged in a logical order starting with the feet and ending with dancing the whole body.

For consistency and ease of orientation the exercises have been numbered continuously from beginning to end in this book. The exercises are grouped by chapter and have been given fun names to infuse a spirit of playfulness and create a comfortable learning environment. It is known that giving concepts easy-to-remember names increases retention. Using the names consistently builds your vocabulary and provides a clear and effective path for your growth.

Guidelines for Doing the Exercises

The value of doing these exercises is in becoming aware of and sensing how you move—*not* trying to stretch or strengthen your muscles. Use the following guidelines when doing the exercises:

Notice Before and After Differences: Take a moment before starting each exercise to sense yourself. This may simply be feeling how you are sitting or standing. Alternatively, you can do a movement or dance a figure—this is like a "before" snapshot. Throughout the exercise, continue to observe any changes in your sensations. At the end of the exercise, take a moment to sense any changes from having done the exercise. If you did a movement or danced a figure at the beginning of the exercise, repeat it again to see how it is different.

Go Slowly and Gently: Go slowly and stay within a comfortable range (i.e., not going to your limit). Reduce your effort and ambition so that your movements become simpler and easier. Focus on *quality*, not quantity or size.

Use Your Awareness: Use the exercises as opportunities to tune into your sensory awareness. Notice *how* you move.

You might ask yourself questions such as: Which of my bones and joints are moving? Am I holding my breath? Where am I initiating the movement from?

Take Frequent Rests: Pause for a short rest between each step of an exercise. Use this time to scan yourself for new sensations and differences. Rests also provide your nervous system with a chance to integrate your learning and a chance to refresh your attention before doing the next step of the exercise.

Experiment: Play with changing aspects of your movement so that each time is a little different. For example, you might vary the speed or trajectory of your movement, initiate from a different place, or change whether you inhale or exhale as you do the movement. Experimenting like this (as opposed to mechanically doing "reps") will speed your learning.

Use Your Hands: If you are unable to sense what or how a part of you is moving, place your hand there. Use your hand for feedback, clarifying your internal sensations and verifying that you are actually doing what you think you are doing.

Use Your Imagination: Thinking of images, visualizing movement in your mind's eye, and imagining movement kinesthetically are great ways to improve how you move. Many of the exercises already employ these techniques. However, feel free to use your own images and visualizations as well.

Chapter 1
Move Like a Champion Fundamentals

Definition of Terms

Agility: The ability to change one's movement (i.e., speed or direction) efficiently at any point. Good range of motion and coordination of the bones and joints are key to having the strength, balance and control necessary for agility.

Alignment: The act of arranging our bones and joints in relationship to each other when sitting, standing and moving.

Bones: The lightweight yet incredibly strong structures that compose our skeleton. Bones function to move, support and protect our bodies. There are 206 bones in the adult human body!

Gravity: The force of attraction that gives weight to things and causes them to fall toward the Earth.

Joint: The moveable or fixed place where two bones come together. There are about 300 joints in the human body!

Proprioception: Sometimes called the *kinesthetic sense,* this is the perception of movement and position of our joints and body parts. Arising primarily from sensory neurons in our muscles, joints and inner ears, we unconsciously depend on proprioception for balance and to coordinate all of our movements.

Sensory Awareness: Paying attention to our sensations. Practicing this awareness allows us to know what we are doing so that we can do and move as we want.

Our Joints

Joints can be divided into three types:

- *Immovable (or fibrous) joints* permit little or no movement (e.g., bones of the skull).
- *Semi-movable (or cartilaginous) joints* are usually made of cartilage and therefore permit some mobility (e.g., intervertebral discs and the pubic symphysis).
- *Highly moveable (or synovial) joints* (e.g., shoulder, hip, knee, etc.)

As dancers, we are most interested in the third type. Highly moveable joints permit a variety of movements and come in many forms (i.e., ball and socket joint, hinge joint, pivot joint, etc.). Every joint has a normal range of motion. Frequently this range is restricted, either due to stiffness (lack of mobility in the joint) or tension (muscle tightness). Some people experience excessive range of motion in their joints, commonly referred to as being hyper-flexible or double-jointed. While this may sound enviable to people who wish they were more flexible, the lack of sufficient support from the ligaments and muscles around a joint with excessive range makes it more vulnerable to injury.

Being that we are one person, everything is connected. Therefore movement in one joint produces movement in the neighboring joints (and usually beyond). For example, motion in the ankle joint while standing results in movement in the knee and the hip joints.

Dynamic Alignment

Alignment is not a fixed position of body parts—it is dynamic, changing from moment to moment. There is always movement in our bodies, even when we are standing or otherwise appear still to the outside world.

To move with ease and efficiency, our bones must be arranged in a way that supports our weight and allows efficient transmission of force (i.e., we must be well aligned). Since everything is connected, an alignment problem in one part of the body effects our whole self. When we are not well aligned, our muscles do the work of our bones. This means those muscles are not available for movement, resulting in looking and feeling stiff.

We call dancing with dynamic alignment "dancing on the bones." This means being poised and able to move in any direction at any moment, whether that be from standing still or when already in motion. Dancing on the bones improves our stability and increases our range of motion, allowing us to move powerfully yet with ease and grace. By becoming aware of how we move, we are able to improve our alignment and dance on our bones.

Chapter 2
Rev Up Your Engine

In our daily lives, we accumulate unnecessary muscular tension and develop little kinks in the way we stand and move. Fortunately, our organism has its own intelligence capable of balancing out and re-establishing harmonious relationships within ourselves. The most effective way to support these organic processes is by expanding our sensory awareness. When we tune in to the messages our bodies are sending—with an attitude of curiosity, rather than one of judgement or correction—we enter a place of rich discovery and learning. Surprisingly, when we stop "trying" to do things with our will, our innate intelligence can begin to find solutions and possibilities for movement we did not even know were possible!

Developing the ability to consciously direct attention to and sense various parts of ourselves is a practice that grows and improves over time. As we become better at this, our movement grows more precise and we gain greater ability to execute our actions as we intend.

The exercises in this chapter are designed to support your sensory awareness practice, as well as stimulate optimal organization by reducing muscular tension and re-establishing more efficient, effortless alignment of the skeleton.

I. MapQuest Yourself

(Sensing Internal Sensations)

Purpose: An introduction to paying attention to your sensations and internally locating various parts of yourself.

Where Used: An excellent way to begin a lesson or to use before and after learning a new (or refining an existing) technique or figure.

Position: Standing (or sitting or lying down).

1. Standing, close your eyes and tune in to the internal sensations of your body. Notice what comes to the forefront of your attention (e.g., a part of your body, a sense of weight, an itch, etc.).

2. Bring your attention to your right foot. Internally sense whether some parts of the sole of your foot make more contact with the floor than other parts? What is the sense of weight like in your foot? What other qualities do you notice (e.g., temperature, length, width, volume, texture, etc.)? Scan various parts of your right foot (e.g., big toe, little toe, top of foot, outside edge of foot, etc.), noticing the places you feel clearly and the places that are more vague in your sensation.

3. Compare your right and left feet. Does one foot seem more clear or more alive in your awareness?

4. Repeat steps 2-3 with one or more parts of yourself (e.g., one hand, one side of your face, one side of your back, etc.).

5. Optional: "Mapquest" your whole self. You can do this systematically, starting at your feet and continuing up yourself to your head, or take your own scenic route. Either way, make sure to compare your right and left sides. You might be surprised to find that the hills, valleys and roadways are a little different on each side.

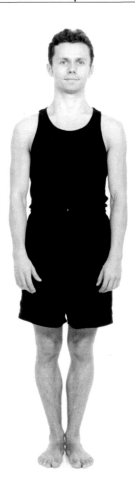

2. Rock Out

(Pushing from the Feet to the Head)

Purpose: To clarify the skeletal connection from foot to head and reduce unnecessary muscular tension for better, more effortless upright posture.

Where Used: A great warm up to prepare for dancing.

Position: Lying on the floor.

1. Lie on the floor with your knees bent and your feet flat on the floor. Have your feet and knees comfortably spread.

2. Gently push the floor with both feet, allowing your pelvis to roll so that your lower back moves toward the floor. Then release, allowing your pelvis to return to neutral.

3. Continue to slowly push and release with the feet, gently rocking your whole self. Begin to track the force as it travels from your feet, through the bones of your legs into your pelvis, and continuing up your spine. What is the response in your head? Play with the rhythm of your rocking, speeding it up and slowing it down again.

4. Experiment with two ways of moving your head. First, allow your chest and neck to be soft so that the force from your feet gently rocks the back of your head on the floor. When you push with your feet, your chin lifts a little away from your chest and when you release, your chin comes closer to your chest. Feel this easy transmission of force through your skeleton.

5. Experiment with a second way of moving your head. Arrange your head in a neutral position. Keeping your face on this same plane, begin to push and release with your feet. The back of your head now slides up and down on the floor. It is as if your spine is a skewer moving up and down relative to your shoulder blades. Each time you push with your feet, your head and neck lengthen out of your chest and shoulders. Sense this feeling of a long spine and neck to recall it when dancing.

6. Alternate between these two ways of moving your head (steps 4-5), clarifying for yourself how they differ.

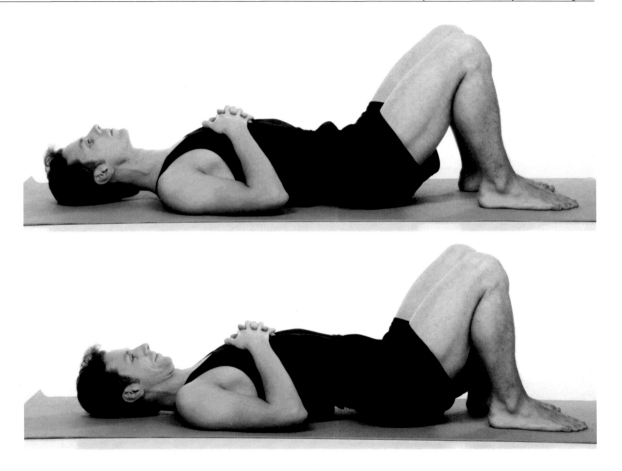

3. Put a Spring in Your Step

(Bouncing on the Heels)

Purpose: To stimulate the natural springiness of our bones and eliminate excess muscular tension. The result is better posture and more efficient transmission of force through the skeleton.

Where Used: Great for a general warm up or when you are tense, nervous or thinking too much.

Position: Standing.

Note: If you have a history of neck or back pain, go very gently. Alternatively, develop your posture and alignment using other exercises, and return to this one at a later date.

1. Stand in a comfortable stance. Lengthen your spine, minimizing the curves of your neck and lower back.

2. Keeping your legs straight, lift both heels off the floor a very small amount. Then let your weight drop, returning your heels to the floor. Repeat this many times in a rhythm that feels good to you. Feel the weight of your skeleton falling through the bones of your legs and heels into the floor. Keep the movement simple and light yet clear.

3. Variations: Repeat step 2 with feet together, on just one leg (and then the other leg), or alternating between right and left legs (as if walking). After doing any of these variations, return to bouncing on both heels.

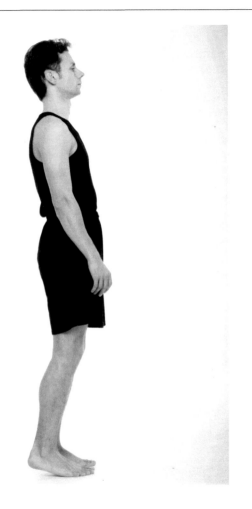 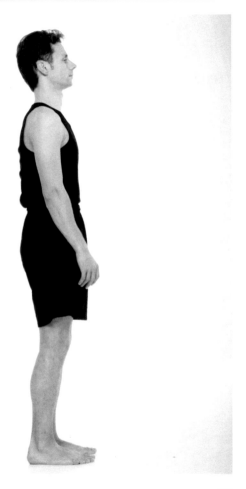

4. Run Baby Run

(Walking and Jogging in Place)

Purpose: To stimulate better upright posture and to energize yourself.

Where Used: A great general warm up.

Position: Standing.

1. Stand comfortably. Take a moment to notice how you are standing. Is there more weight on one foot? How long does your spine feel? How does your head rest on top of your spine?

2. Begin to walk in place, changing weight from one foot to the other. Allow the rest of yourself to move naturally as you change weight. Imagine that your spine lengthens in both directions as you walk—your head floating toward the ceiling and your tailbone dropping toward the floor. Feel how your weight goes into the floor on each step.

3. Stop a moment and notice how you stand now. Does anything feel different from before?

4. Start to jog in place in a relaxed way. Make sure to slightly lift your free foot from the floor in between weight changes. Sense how weight travels through you into the floor. Reduce your effort so that the movement is simple and light.

5. Observe your sensations. Has standing upright become easier in any way?

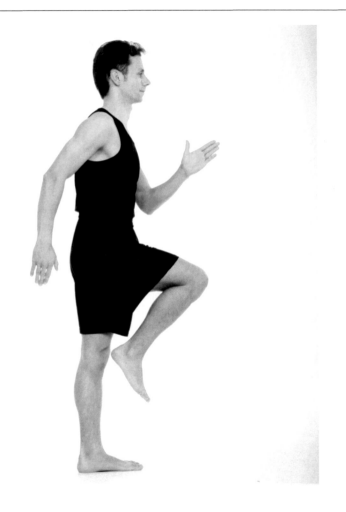
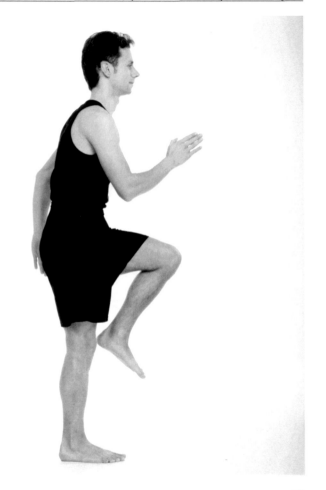

Chapter 3
Feet and Ankles

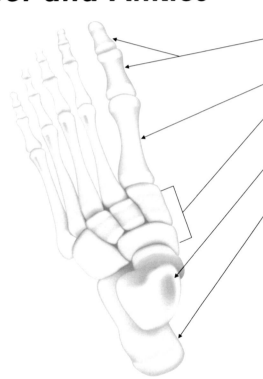

Bones and Joints of the Feet and Ankles

There are 26 bones and 33 joints in each foot and ankle! The following are the most useful to know as a dancer.

Phalanges: The bones of the toes. Analogous to our hands, there are two phalanges in the big toe and three in each of the other toes.

Metatarsals: The five long bones between the ankle and toes.

Tarsals: The five irregular-shaped bones that form the arch of the foot—the cuboid, navicular and three cuneiform bones.

Talus: Also called the *ankle bone,* this is the uppermost bone in the foot and forms the lower part of the ankle joint.

Calcaneus: The heel bone.

Ankle Joint: A hinge joint between the talus and the bones of the lower leg (i.e., tibia and fibula).

Functions of the Feet and Ankles

When upright, our feet and ankles are our base of support, and therefore are key to our balance, stability and mobility. The human foot and ankle are brilliantly designed for two main functions—support and movement.

The feet and ankles carry the entire weight of the body and act as shock absorbers (in a one-mile run, they sustain several tons of pressure). The majority of support comes from the outside of the foot (i.e., the fourth and fifth metatarsals and toes, and the bones on the outside of the foot, all the way to the ankle joint).

The feet and ankles also propel us through space, nimbly adapting to the various surfaces on which we move. Propulsion comes primarily from the inside of the foot (i.e., the first three metatarsals and toes, and all the bones on the inside of the foot, all the way to the ankle joint).

Increasing our awareness enables us to utilize the full range of possibilities in our feet and ankles!

5. Get to Know Your Feet and Ankles

Remove your shoes and sit on a chair. Bend your right leg and rest the right ankle on your left knee. Locate the various bones of your right foot and the ankle joint (then on your left foot, if desired):

- **Calcaneus (Heel):** This bone is easy to feel at the back of the foot, and less directly through the thick pad on the bottom of the heel.

- **Talus (Ankle Bone) and Ankle Joint:** The talus sits just above the calcaneus and below the knobby bumps of the ankle. The top surface of the talus and the bottom surfaces of the knobby bumps form the ankle joint. Gently bend and straighten the ankle to feel this joint in action.

- **Tarsals:** The tarsals are in front of the ankle, and can be most easily felt from the top of the foot. Experiment with the movements the joints between the tarsals, talus and calcaneus allow, such as rolling the foot inward (inversion) and outward (eversion), and moving the foot side to side.

- **Metatarsals (Foot Bones):** Touch the top of the foot and feel each of the five metatarsals that connect to your toes.

- **Phalanges (Toes)**

  1. Use your hands to gently bend all your toes down (as if to touch the sole of the foot), and then up (as if to touch the top of the foot).

  2. Locate the joint at the base of the big toe in the ball of the foot. This is where the end of the first metatarsal meets the big toe. With one hand on this joint and the other holding the middle of your big toe, gently bend and extend the joint. This will move the big toe down (toward the sole of the foot) and up (toward the top of the foot). Do this several times, finding an easy range of mobility in this joint.

  3. Repeat step 2 with each of the remaining four toes of the right foot.

  4. Stand and notice the sensations in each foot. Does the right foot feel different than the left?

6. Grow a Shoe Size
(Spreading the Feet with a Ball)

Purpose: To increase the flexibility of the feet and ankles and improve balance.

Where Used: A great warm up for the feet.

Position: Standing.

Props: Tennis or pinky ball.

1. Remove your shoes. Stand in a comfortable stance, with weight on both feet.

2. Begin to shift your weight from front to back. Notice the parts of your feet and how they make contact with the floor as the weight shifts.

3. Now place a tennis (or pinky) ball under the ball of the right foot. Keeping the heel on the floor, let your foot drape over the ball. Begin to roll the foot over the ball from side to side, opening and stretching the metatarsals.

4. Then, with most of your weight on the foot, roll the ball forward and back lengthwise along the sole of your foot, enjoying a massage that spreads the foot in all directions.

5. With the ball under the front of the foot, shoot the ball out from under your toes. Do this a few times seeing how much you are able to control the aim and distance of your shooting.

6. Repeat steps 3 and 4 with the left foot.

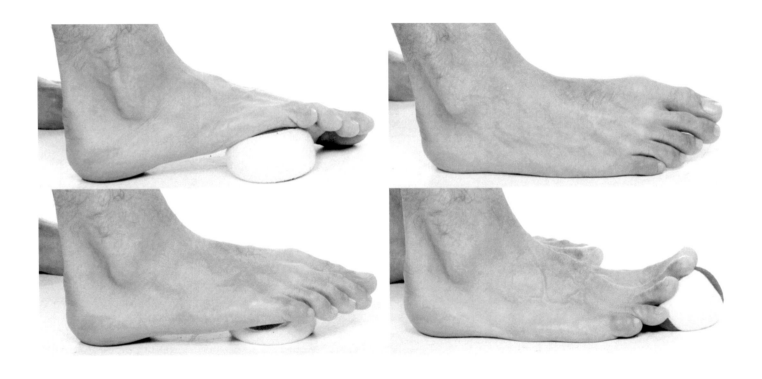

7. Feet with Attitude

(Shaping the Free Foot)

Purpose: To differentiate the movement of the feet and ankles for increased strength and flexibility, as well as more precise and expressive use of the feet.

Where Used: Everywhere for nice articulation of the feet in all dances.

Position: Sitting.

1. Remove your shoes and sit on the front edge of a chair. Interlace your hands under your right thigh and hold the leg so that the right foot is hanging free from the floor.

2. Bend the right ankle (top of the foot gets closer to the shin) and then straighten it (top of the foot moves away from the shin). Slowly alternate between bending and straightening the ankle several times. Feel how the ankle moves—how one side lengthens as the opposite bends.

3. Now give your foot attitude by pointing the toes as you straighten the ankle. Think of lengthening the top of your foot, not squeezing or grabbing with your toes.

4. Again hold under your right thigh so that the foot is in the air. Begin drawing clockwise circles with your right big toe (although the focus is on your big toe, the whole foot circles). Switch to thinking that your little toe draws the circles. Continue to play with thinking of different parts of your foot drawing the circles, noticing how this affects the movement.

5. Reverse the direction of the circles. Go slowly, finding the points of the circle at which your foot and ankle create these shapes used in dancing: heel lead, inside edge for Latin and Tango (as well as brushing actions), and pointing the foot.

6. Repeat steps 1-5 with your left foot.

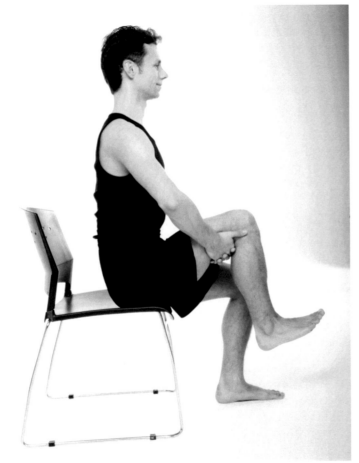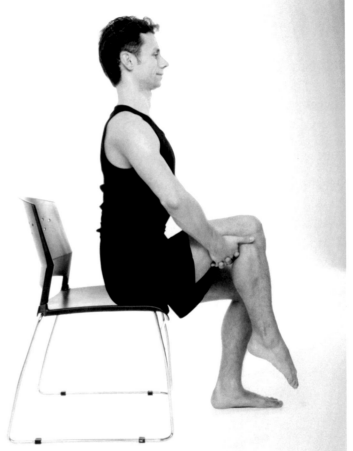

8. Guitar String Feet

(Using the Five Lines of the Feet)

Purpose: To utilize all five lines of the feet for increased stability, strength and balance. and to find the most efficient way to roll weight through the feet.

Where Used: Every forward and back walk.

Position: Sitting and standing.

1. Remove your shoes and stand with weight primarily on the right foot. Begin to shift weight forward and back on the foot. Notice how and where your weight naturally rolls (e.g., more to the inside or outside edge, in a straight or curving line, etc.).

2. Sit on a chair and bring your right foot to rest on your left knee. Using your left thumb and index finger, take hold of the end of your right little toe. Gently lengthen and then begin to turn the toe around its axis. Feel the entire line of the toe and its metatarsal (i.e., the guitar string). Repeat this with each of the remaining toes on your right foot.

3. Stand again with weight primarily on your right foot. Notice any differences from before. Shift your weight to the outside edge of the right heel and begin moving your weight forward and back along the line (guitar string) of the little toe. Repeat this with each of the remaining toes on your right foot.

4. Repeat steps 1-3 with your left foot.

5. Slowly walk forward around the room. Notice which guitar string the weight rolls through on each of your feet—are they the same or different?

6. Play with rolling the weight through different strings as you walk. While rolling through all strings of the guitar, emphasize rolling through an imaginary sixth string between the lines of the big toe and second toe. Notice how the last thing to peel off the floor with each step are these two toes.

7. Repeat steps 5 and 6 walking backward.

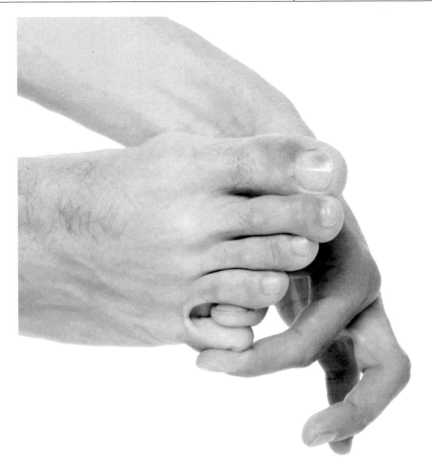

9. Barbie Feet

(Standing on the Platform*)

Purpose: To be able to use the ball of the foot and have stability while rising.

Where Used: Rise and fall, Samba bounce and swing bounce.

Position: Sitting and standing.

* *Platform:* A nickname for standing on the toes and frontmost part of the ball of the foot with the heel high off the floor. Dancers stand on the platform when using toe footwork.

1. Remove your shoes and sit on the front edge of a chair. Interlace your hands under your right thigh and hold the leg so that your right foot is hanging free from the floor.

2. Slowly bend and straighten your right ankle joint several times (i.e., top of the foot moves toward, then away from the shin).

3. Keeping your ankle joint quiet, slowly bend your toes down and then lift them up. As you repeat this several times, notice if some toes move more than others or if one toe leads the rest. Gradually find how to move all your toes equally and in smooth coordination.

4. Bend your ankle joint in combination with bending your toes down (i.e., bend the ankle while curling the toes under). Return to neutral and repeat several times. Bend both the ankle and toes simultaneously, making this into one coordinated movement.

5. Now do the opposite—straighten the ankle joint while lifting the toes. Return to neutral and repeat several times. Notice this is the platform position of the foot, very much like the shape of a Barbie's feet (i.e., as if wearing high heel shoes).

6. Repeat steps 2-5 with the left foot.

7. Stand with weight on your left foot. Lift your right heel as high as possible, bending at the base of the toes (i.e., standing on the platform of the foot). Have most of your weight between the base of the big toe and second toe (i.e., the sixth guitar string).

Observe how your ankle joint is extended and forms a straight line with the shin. Notice that your toes form a 90-degree angle with the metatarsals. Slowly lower your right heel, tracking how these angles change. Repeat a few times.

8. Repeat step 7 standing on the right foot, lifting the left heel.

9. Stand with weight on both feet. Shift your weight forward (toward the toes), gradually lifting both heels from the floor, until you arrive standing on the platform. Lower, then repeat a few times. As you do this, observe the changing angles of your joints.

10. Remaining on the platform of both feet, begin to walk around the room. You might imagine you are tip-toeing as if to sneak around without anyone hearing you.

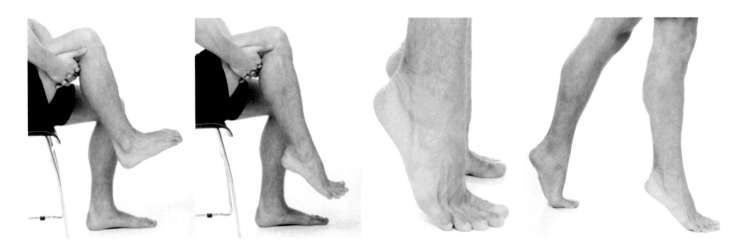

Top Pointers for the Feet and Ankles

1. Spread your feet so that they are wide, flexible and stable (*Grow a Shoe Size*).

2. When shifting weight to or through the front of your foot, direct the weight between the base of your big toe and second toe (*Guitar String Feet*).

3. On steps with *toe* footwork, stand on the platform of the foot (*Barbie Feet*). The toes are spread and long on the floor, and the heel is raised high.

4. When pointing your feet, stretch your toes long—do not squeeze or grip them (*Feet with Attitude*).

5. When pointing your foot forward, the inside of the foot faces upward. When pointing your foot back, the inside of the foot faces downward (*Feet with Attitude*).

6. When pointing your foot to the side, showcase the top of your foot, keeping slight pressure on the inside edge of your big toe and your ankle angled slightly toward the floor (*Feet with Attitude*).

7. To turn out your feet, start in parallel and think of turning your heels *in* rather than your toes out. This rotates your femurs in their hip sockets, creating true turnout.

8. Remember that your foot is an extension of your leg, not a separate entity. Allow the movements of your feet and legs to be connected.

Chapter 4
Knees and Legs

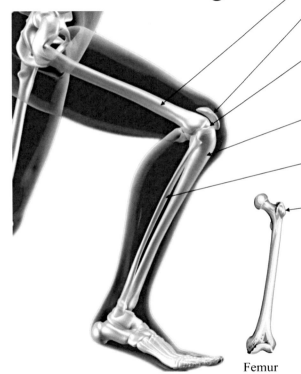

Femur

Bones and Joints of the Knees and Legs

- **Femur:** The thigh bone.

- **Patella:** The floating bone at the front of the knee joint, also called the *knee cap*.

- **Knee Joint:** The largest and most complicated joint in the body comprised of three bones—the femur (above), the tibia (below) and the patella (in front). It is primarily a hinge joint.

- **Tibia:** The larger bone of the lower leg, also called the *shin bone*. The tibia is the primary weight bearer of the lower leg.

- **Fibula:** The smaller of the two lower leg bones, also called the *calf bone*.

- **Greater Trochanter:** The large bony protuberance on the outside of the femur, just below the head of the femur.

Functions of the Knees and Legs

Our legs are a primary source of power for propelling us through space. The quadricep muscles at the front of the thighs are some of the largest in the body. While the use of our legs is intimately connected with the pelvis and the feet, our legs also have tremendous freedom to move independently from pelvis.

The knee is primarily a hinge joint that bends forward and straightens. The knees are not built for rotation when weight bearing and are vulnerable to injury from torquing. Therefore it is important to use the knees as they are meant to move and to develop smooth coordination between the knee, ankle and hip joints. In addition to preventing strain and injury, the better coordinated the knees are with these other joints, the more powerful and graceful our movement will be.

10. Get to Know Your Knees and Legs

Sitting on a chair, cross your right leg over the left in a comfortable manner. Locate the following (then repeat on the left leg, if desired):

- **Patella (Knee Cap):** Feel its outline at the front of your knee.

- **Tibia (Shin Bone):** Feel along the front of the leg from just below the patella down to the bony knob on the inside of your ankle.

- **Knee Joint:** Feel the sides of your leg at about patella height. This is where the tibia meets the bottom of your femur, and along with the patella, forms your knee joint. Gently bend and straighten your leg to feel the knee joint in action.

- **Fibula (Calf Bone):** Feel on the outside of your lower leg just below the knee for a round bony bump—this is the top end of your fibula. Then feel its bottom end —the bump on the outside of your ankle.

- **Femur (Thigh Bone):** Now stand and place your palm on the outside of your right hip where your leg meets your torso. Slowly rotate your leg in and out. Feel for a large bony bump moving forward and back underneath your hand. This is the uppermost part of your femur (i.e., greater trochanter) before it bends inward to the hip joint.

From there, palpate down the outside of your thigh, following the length of your femur. Just above the knee you will find a bony bump (with a corresponding bump on the inside side). This is the bottom end of your femur.

11. Smooth Operator

(Coordinating Hip, Knee, Ankle and Toe Joints)

Purpose: To create smooth and powerful lowering and rising by moving the hip, knee ankle and toe joints in harmony.

Where Used: Everywhere, especially in Smooth and Standard, Bolero and Samba.

Position: Sitting on floor, then standing.

1. Sit on the floor with your legs long and lean back on your hands. Initiate drawing your right leg up by flexing your right ankle. Continue to bend your right leg until the bottom of the right foot is on the floor (i.e., your foot is "standing"). Then flex your ankle to initiate bringing your right leg back down. As you straighten your leg, think of lengthening through your heel. Repeat this a few times, starting each movement by bending your ankle. Feel the relationship between your ankle, knee and hip joints, making it smoother each time.

2. Repeat step 1 with the left leg.

3. Standing, begin to bend both your knees. Notice how the ankle and hip joints bend as well. Observe that the angle between your lower legs and tops of your feet decreases as you lower. Slowly straighten your legs and then repeat. Continue until you have a clear sense of how all three joints work together for effortless bending and straightening.

4. Slowly rise onto the platforms of both feet. Feel how this movement is happening almost entirely in your "toe" joints (i.e., where your metatarsals meet your phalanges). At your highest point, notice that your metatarsals are at right angles with your toes. Slowly lower to your normal standing height, and repeat a few times.

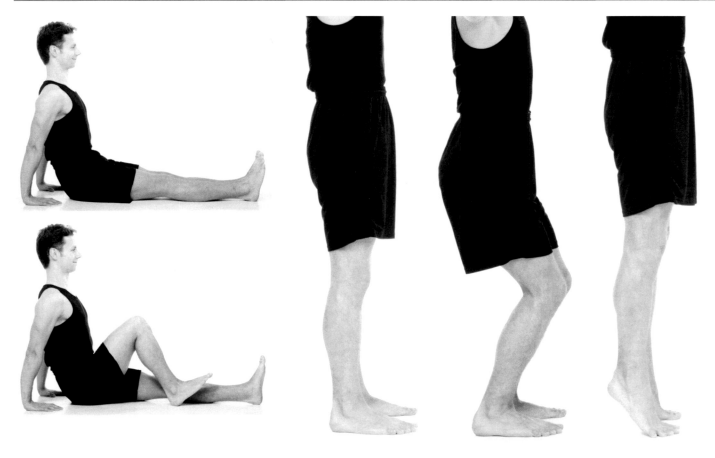

12. Total Eclipse of the Toes

(Tracking the Knees)

Purpose: To learn how to track the knees over the feet safely and efficiently.

Where Used: Whenever bending and straightening the knees.

Position: Standing.

1. Stand with your feet slightly apart. Begin to bend and straighten your knees, being aware of how the shin bones travel forward over the feet. Which toe(s) do your knees track over?

2. Bring your attention to your right leg and knee. Begin to slowly bend and straighten the right leg, consciously tracking the right knee over the fifth toe (i.e., baby toe). Go very gently. Notice how this feels in terms of ease and stability.

3. Repeat step 2 with each of the remaining four toes. Then find how to track between first and second toes (i.e., the imaginary sixth guitar string) for the greatest ease, comfort and stability. To test that you are doing this correctly, glance down and see if your knee covers your toes. If you are able to see your toes, your knee is probably tracking too far to the inside or outside of your foot.

4. Repeat steps 2 and 3 with your left knee.

5. Bend and straighten both knees simultaneously, tracking over the line between the first and second toes.

Note: If you have knee injuries, go very gently with this exercise, especially tracking the knees over the third through fifth toes. You may want to just imagine tracking the knees over these toes.

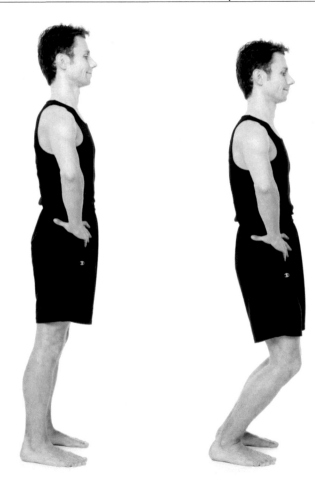

13. Tony Heelney

(Coordinating the Toe, Knee and Ankle Joints)

Purpose: For smooth and graceful lowering from the platform position.

Where Used: Whenever lowering from an up position. For example: Count 3 in Waltz, counts 1 and 2 in Samba, the end of the first Quick in Bolero.

Position: Standing.

1. Stand with feet together. Rise onto the platforms of your feet (i.e., toes).

2. Begin to lower with control, first bending your knees and then returning your heels to the floor. Once your heels are on the floor, continue bending the knees into a lowered position (e.g., in Waltz). To guide you in this sequence, simply say the name of the great dance teacher Mr. Tony Heelney (i.e., toe-knee-heel-knee).

3. Repeat steps 1 and 2 several times.

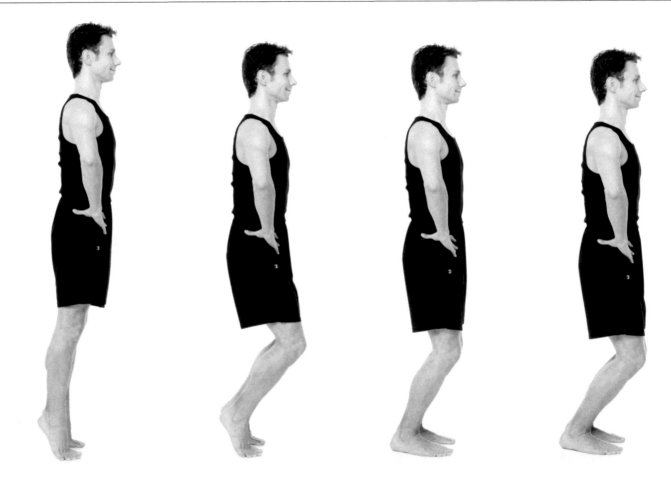

14. Knee on a String

(Moving the Whole Leg)

Purpose: To travel forward in the Rhythm and Latin dances with balance and power.

Where Used: Every forward step in the Rhythm and Latin dances.

Position: Standing.

Props: String, rope or yoga strap.

1. Stand with your weight on a straight right leg. Tie a string (or similar item) around your left knee.

2. Have a partner pull the string, slowly moving your left knee forward. Allow your left knee to move as much as possible *before* peeling your left foot off the floor—first the heel, then the ball, and finally the toes. Since your knee is connected to your upper and lower leg, your whole leg moves forward to take the step. Repeat this a few times.

3. For contrast, tie the string to your left foot. Have your partner gently pull the string, causing you to take a forward step with your foot leading the way. Moving from the foot like this is a common mistake.

4. Return the string to your left knee. Again, have your partner pull the string, and move your whole leg to take a forward step (delaying the movement of the left foot). Compare this to moving from your foot.

5. Repeat steps 2-4 standing on your left foot with the string tied around your right knee.

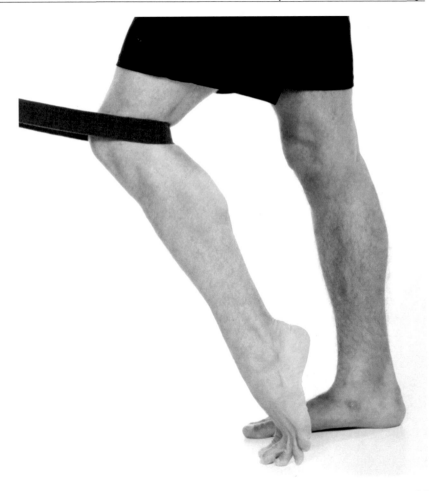

Top Pointers for the Knees and Legs

1. Keep your knees soft, not locked.

2. When bending your knees, track them over your first and second toes—that is, your imaginary guitar string (*Guitar String Feet, Total Eclipse of the Toes*).

3. Bend your knees only as far as you can maintain a neutral alignment of your pelvis and spine.

4. When standing, any movement in the knee joint necessitates movement in the ankle and hip joints. Therefore, when bending and straightening your standing leg, smoothly coordinate all three joints (*Smooth Operator*).

5. In the Smooth and Standard dances, knee bending is for the purpose of lowering and creating the power to move (*Tony Heelney*).

6. When lowering from an "up" position in the Smooth and Standard dances and in Samba, begin to bend your knees before your heels reach the floor. Once your heels are down, continue bending your knees (*Tony Heelney*).

7. Generally, in the Rhythm and Latin dances, the knee of the free leg should face the same direction as the knee of the standing leg after a side step is taken.

8. When you think of moving your leg, you will go. It is as if your legs are the wheels of a car—when they are working, your car moves.

Chapter 5
Pelvis and Hip Joints

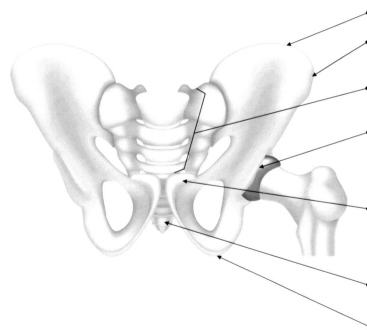

Bones and Joints of the Pelvis

Pelvis: The bowl-shaped structure connecting the spine and legs, comprised of two hip bones, the sacrum and coccyx.

Iliac Crest: The top edge of the pelvis.

ASIS (Anterior Superior Iliac Spine): The front edge of each hip bone.

Sacrum: The large triangular bone at the base of the spine which is both a part of the spine and pelvis.

Hip Joint: The ball-and-socket joint formed by the concave socket in each hip bone and the round head of each femur bone. The hip joints are located at the sides of the pelvis and are angled slightly downward.

Pubic Bone: The frontmost of the three bones that fuse to form each hip bone. Pubic bone is also casually used as a synonym for the *pubic symphysis*—the place where the two hip bones join at the lower front of the pelvis.

Coccyx: The bottom segment of our spine, also known as the *tailbone.*

Ischial Tuberosity: The two protuberances on the bottom of the pelvis that we sit on, also known as the *sit bones.*

Functions of the Pelvis and Hip Joints

The pelvis is the glue that connects our upper and lower body, and therefore is key to our posture and coordination. It serves as a relay station for the forces traveling up from the legs and for the weight of the upper body traveling in the opposite direction. Our center of gravity and the strong muscles of our core are located in the pelvis, making it the prime initiator of our movement and source of power. The hip joints allow a huge range of motion—forward and back (i.e., extension and flexion), side to side (i.e., abduction and adduction), and rotation (i.e., internal and external rotation). This gives our pelvis and legs the freedom to move together or separately. While everyone's hip sockets are different (i.e., location, angle and depth), the average external rotation of the hip joint (i.e., turnout) is about 45 degrees. The amount of internal rotation is significantly less.

The pelvic floor is the name for the set of muscles that span the bottom opening of the pelvis. Often overlooked, the pelvic floor is intimately connected with the use of our core muscles and in providing support for upright posture.

Increasing our awareness of our pelvis and hip joints improves our alignment, our ability to move powerfully, our partner connection, leg swing and more!

15. Get to Know Your Pelvis and Hip Joints

Locate various parts of your pelvis and hip joints:

- **Pelvic Landmarks:** In either sitting or standing, locate the sacrum, coccyx, iliac crest, ASIS, pubic bone and ischial tuberosities (sitting bones). An alternative way to feel the sitting bones is to sit on a firm chair and gently tilt the pelvis forward and back.

- **Hip Joint:** When standing, find the indentation on one side of your buttocks (toward the outside and bottom) and place your palm there. Begin turning your femur in and out and feel the movement under your hand. This is the back of your hip joint.

  Now sit on a chair and hug your leg to your chest. Move your leg with your hands, exploring the range of motion in your hip joint. If desired, repeat on the other side.

- **Pelvic Floor:** In either sitting or standing, feel the pelvic floor muscles by thinking of an octopus contracting and moving up. Other helpful images for finding these muscles are zipping up a tight pair of pants or stopping the flow of urine.

16. Don't Get Tipsy
(Neutral Positioning of the Pelvis)

Purpose: To feel the forward and back range of motion of the pelvis and then identify "neutral"—the most balanced and aligned position for moving.

Where Used: Everywhere.

Position: Standing.

1. Standing with knees slightly bent, place your hands on your hips. Imagine that your pelvis is a bowl or large drinking glass filled with liquid.

2. Using your hands, begin to tilt the bowl of the pelvis forward and back like a swing. Notice how the liquid sloshes (and perhaps spills out) as you do this.

3. Gradually decrease the size of the movement, finding a place in the middle where the liquid in your bowl is level—that is a neutral position of the pelvis.

4. Some markers of a neutral pelvis are that the abdomen is slightly lifted without squeezing and the tailbone hangs softly, neither tucked under nor tipped up. Also, the crease between the butt and thigh is parallel to the floor. You might imagine holding a pencil in this crease.

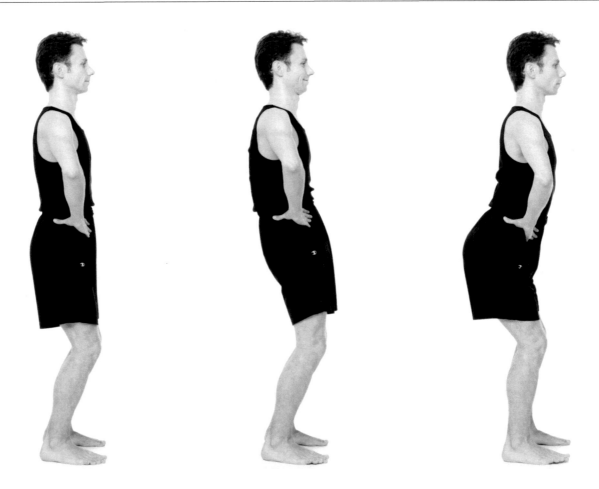

17. Turn on Your Headlights

(Neutral Positioning of the Pelvis)

Purpose: Another way to find the neutral position of the pelvis.

Where Used: Everywhere.

Position: Walking.

1. In standing, make soft fists with your hands. Place the little finger side of each fist on the front of its hip bone (i.e., the ASIS). Feel the contact your fists make and notice the angle of the hip bones. Are they pointed straight forward or are they a little up or down?

2. Imagine you are a car and your fists and hip bones are your headlights. Just like the headlights of a car, you want your lights to shine forward on the road in front of you. Find the neutral alignment of your pelvis in which your headlights are directed forward and start walking.

3. As you continue walking forward, tip the top of your pelvis backward (reducing the curve in your lower back) so that your headlights shine a bit upward. Observe what it is like to walk with your pelvis in this position. Then tip the top of your pelvis forward (increasing the arch in your lower back) so that your headlights shine down toward the floor. Notice how this effects your walking.

4. Once again, shine your headlights directly forward with your pelvis in neutral.

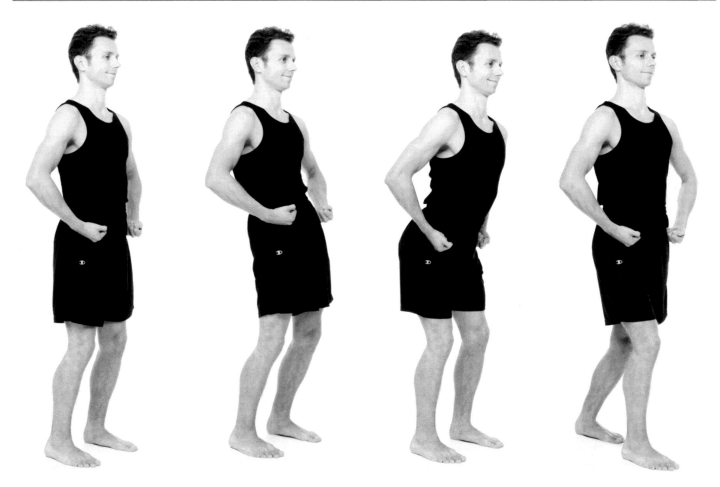

18. Rock the Boat

(Tilting the Pelvis Side to Side)

Purpose: Tilting the pelvis side to side while keeping it in a neutral forward and back alignment.

Where Used: All dances with Latin hip action and sway, as well as Bolero hip lifts.

Position: Standing.

1. Stand with weight on a straight left leg. Your right leg is to the side without weight except for slight pressure on the inside edge of the ball of the foot.

2. Gently lift and lower the right side of your pelvis while keeping your spine vertical. Repeat several times, noticing that the pelvis rotates around the head of the left femur, which remains more or less still. Notice the action of lifting the right side of your pelvis is like a Bolero hip lift, and lowering it is like doing Latin hip action. While doing this, keep your weight toward the inside edge of your left foot.

3. Gently tilt your pelvis to the left. This time, tilt your whole spine and head with the pelvis. Notice that this is essentially what you do when creating sway.

4. Repeat steps 1-3 standing on the right leg.

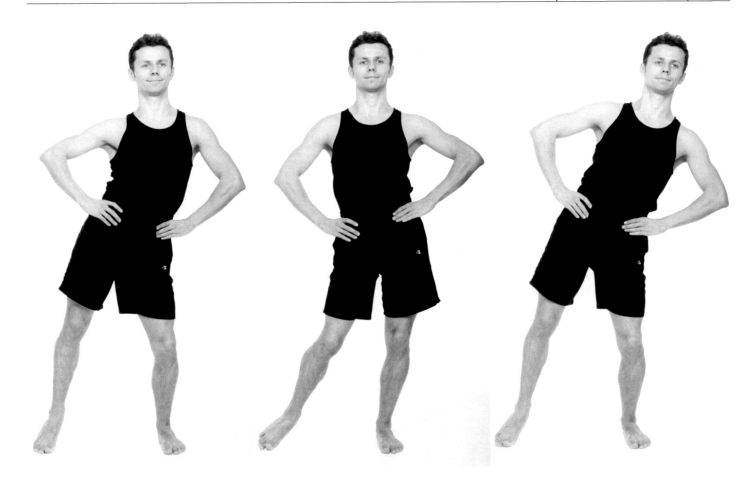

19. Get a Leg Up
(Swinging the Leg with a Neutral, Level Pelvis)

Purpose: To learn how to swing the legs freely in the hip joints while the pelvis stays in neutral.

Where Used: All forward and back steps. All side steps without sway or Latin hip action.

Position: Standing on a step or prop.

Props: A step or a thick book, yoga block or similar object that elevates you an inch or more off the floor. If none of these are available, do the exercise with one shoe off.

1. Stand with the right foot on a step or prop so the left foot hangs free from the floor. It is best to stand near a wall, rail or back of a chair that can be used for balance if necessary. Make sure the right and left sides of your pelvis are level in spite of standing elevated on one leg.

2. Slowly start to swing your left leg a little forward and back in its hip joint while keeping your pelvis in neutral. Place a hand on either the front or back of your pelvis to feel whether your pelvis remains in neutral or if it tilts as your leg swings. Also, notice that the relationship between your left leg and pelvis is changing (i.e., the leg alternately comes closer to the front and then the back of your pelvis). Meanwhile, the relationship between your standing right leg and pelvis stays the same.

3. For comparison, allow your pelvis to tilt with the left leg as it swings. Now the relationship between your standing right leg and pelvis is also changing. Then return to keeping your pelvis in neutral as you swing the leg.

4. Repeat steps 1-3 standing on the left foot, swinging the right leg.

5. Stand with the right foot on the step or prop again. Swing the left leg a small amount to the side and return (the left foot stays parallel to the right). Repeat several times, keeping your pelvis both level and in neutral. Notice that the relationship between your pelvis and standing right leg remains the same, while the relationship with the left leg changes.

6. For comparison, allow your pelvis to go with the left leg as it moves to the side (i.e., the left side of your pelvis will lift).

how the relationship between your standing right leg and pelvis changes now—the pelvis tilts around the head of the right femur, changing the angle between the right leg and the pelvis. Then return to keeping your pelvis level as you swing the leg to the side.

7. Repeat steps 5 and 6 standing on the left foot and swinging the right leg.

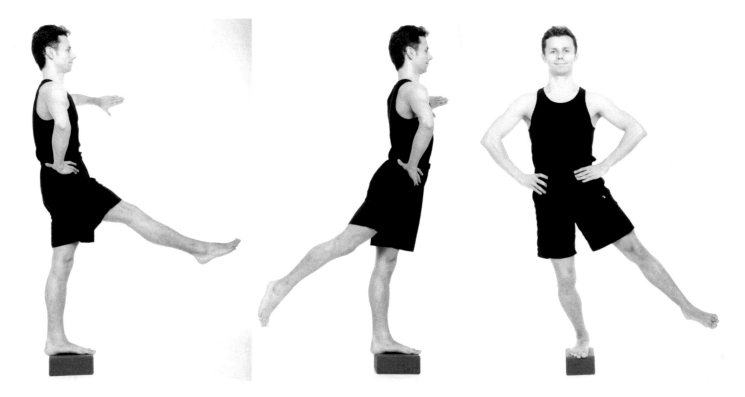

20. Heel Compass
(Connecting Heel to Hip Joint to Torso)

Purpose: Using the heel of the free or standing leg to help direct the entire body to turn.

Where Used: Back steps with turn and some pivots (free leg). Spot turns and swivels (standing leg).

Position: Standing.

Heel Compass for Free Leg

1. Stand with weight on your left foot. Begin to swing your right leg back, commencing turn to the left (as if dancing the back half of a left turning box in Waltz).

2. In coordination with the turning of your pelvis, aim your right heel to the right. You might imagine your heel is the needle of a compass, pointing the way. Notice how turning your heel internally rotates the bones of the right leg. Sense how the head of your right femur "hooks" into its hip joint, connecting the leg to the pelvis.

3. For contrast, begin to swing your right leg back again. This time, turn your pelvis without thinking about turning your right heel (or even allow your right foot to turn out slightly). Notice how this hinders your ability to turn to the left. Then return to swinging the leg back, thinking of the right heel as your compass.

4. Repeat steps 1-3 stepping back on the left foot, commencing turn to the right.

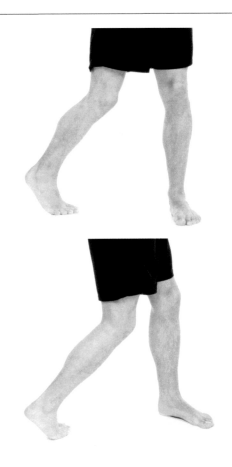

Heel Compass for Standing Leg

1. Stand with weight on your right foot and dance a spot turn (switch turn) to the right. Stepping your left foot forward and across, transfer weight onto the left foot and turn your left heel 1/2 turn to the right. Think of quickly pointing your heel compass in the opposite direction.

2. Replace weight to your right foot and take three walks forward —left, right, left.

3. Dance a spot turn to the left. Stepping your right foot forward and across, transfer your weight onto the right foot and turn your right heel 1/2 turn left (to point in the opposite direction). Notice if thinking of turning your heel improves the crispness and ease of your turn.

4. Replace weight to the left foot and take three walks forward— right, left, right.

5. Repeat steps 1-4 several times.

6. For contrast, repeat steps 1-4 without thinking about turning your heels. See how this changes your turning. Then return to using your heel compasses to aid your turns.

21. Bottle Brush

(Differentiating the Pelvis and Femur)

Purpose: Clarifying when the pelvis turns and when the leg (femur) turns.

Where Used: Whenever turning.

Position: Standing at a wall, rail or table.

1. Imagine each of the concave hip sockets of your pelvis is a drinking glass (the glasses are turned to match the orientation of your hip sockets). Then imagine each of your femurs is a bottle brush, the kind used to clean glasses. The length of the femur is the handle and the head of the femur is the brush. To clean the glasses of your hip sockets, you may move the glass (pelvis) or the bottle brush (femur).

2. Stand on your right leg (if helpful, use a wall, rail or table for balance). Begin to turn your pelvis a little right and left, keeping your right femur still. Feel how your glass turns around the brush.

3. Standing on your right leg again, start to turn your left femur a little in and out, keeping your pelvis still. Sense how you now turn the brush (of your free leg) while the glass remains stationary.

4. Shift your weight slightly forward on your right foot. Begin to turn your right femur a little in and out (turning on the ball of the foot) while keeping your pelvis still. Now you are turning the brush of your standing leg within the glass of your right hip socket.

5. Repeat steps 2-4 standing on your left leg.

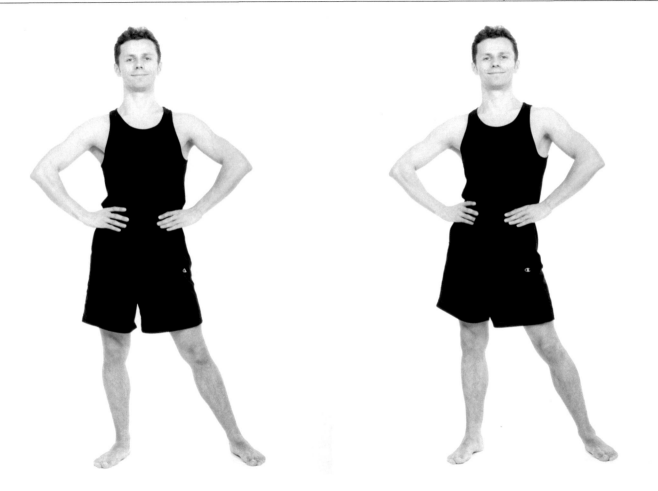

22. Orgasmic Figure Eights

(Using the Heads of the Femurs in Latin Hip Action)

Purpose: To clarify how the heads of the femurs move in relationship to the pelvis to create Latin hip action.

Where Used: Latin hip action.

Position: Standing.

1. Stand with your feet in a comfortable stance. Begin doing figure eights with your pelvis. Observe how your pelvis moves and where the weight is on your feet.

2. Sense the location of the heads of your femurs internally. Begin to do figure eights again, this time thinking of drawing them with the heads of your femurs. First move the head of one femur forward and circle it to the back (without going too far out to the side), then repeat on the other side. Notice how your pelvis moves differently from before. Is there a difference in the quality or size? Generally the movement will be a little smaller yet smoother and more connected.

3. Repeat step 2 again, paying attention to how the weight moves on your feet. Keep weight toward the inside edges of the feet. Allow your weight to shift from the front to the back of your standing foot in coordination with the stirring movement of the head of your femur.

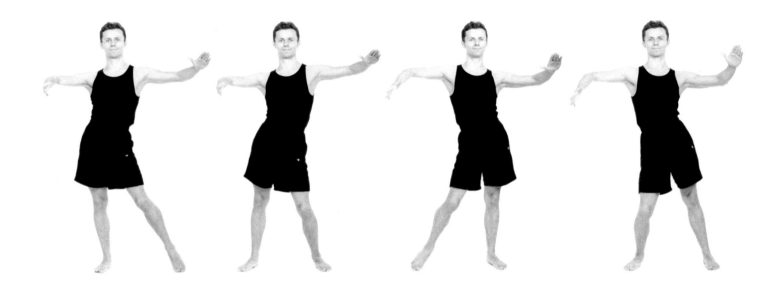

Top Pointers for the Pelvis and Hip Joints

1. Find and maintain neutral positioning of your pelvis for stability and balance (*Don't Get Tipsy* and *Turn on Your Headlights*).

2. Support the neutral positioning of your pelvis by slightly engaging your abdominal muscles.

3. Allow your moving leg to swing freely from the hip joint (*Get a Leg Up*), tracking the leg under your pelvis (rather than swinging it wide).

4. Remember that your hip joints allow your pelvis to turn independently or together with your legs (*Bottle Brush*).

5. When dancing figure eights, concentrate on moving from your hip joints, *not* moving the entire pelvis (*Orgasmic Figure Eights*).

6. The pelvis is a prime initiator of movement—remember to use its power!

Chapter 6
Spine

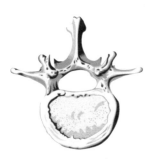

Lumbar Vertebra
(top view)

Bones and Regions of the Spine

Vertebra: An individual bone of the spinal column, divided by intervertebral discs. There are 24 vertebra in our spine (plus the sacrum and coccyx).

Cervical Spine: The seven vertebra of the neck.

Thoracic Spine: The twelve vertebra of the mid and upper back to which the ribs attach.

Lumbar Spine: The five large vertebra at the bottom of the spine.

Sacrum: The large triangular bone at the base of the spine. The sacrum articulates with the last lumbar vertebra (above), the coccyx (below), and each hip bone (to the sides).

Coccyx: The bottom segment of our spine, also known as the *tailbone*.

Functions of the Spine

The central axis of our body, the spine connects our pelvis and head and supports us in being vertical. The joints between our vertebra allow for a wide range of movement—they are able to turn and bend in all directions (forward, back and side).

While people often talk about having a "straight" spine, the reality is that our spine has curves—the lumbar and cervical spine curve inward, while the sacrum and coccyx, and thoracic spine curve outward. These are essential shock absorbers for our movement. Therefore we want to maintain the gentle curves of our spine.

Being aware of how we use our spine directly benefits our posture, flexibility, shaping, turning and partner connection.

23. Get to Know Your Spine

Locate the following parts of your spine. Alternatively, do this with a partner.

- **Sacrum and Coccyx (Tailbone)**: Gently feel your coccyx and the outline of your sacrum.

- **Lumbar Spine**: Feel the bony processes of your lower back vertebrae.

- **Thoracic Spine**: Continue moving up your spine (as much as comfortable), feeling the vertebrae in your mid and upper back.

- **Cervical Spine**: Feel the vertebrae at the back of your neck.

Three Planes of Spinal Movement

Movement of the spine can be divided into three planes.

1. **Forward and Back:** Bending forward (i.e., flexing) and arching backward (i.e., extending).

2. **Side:** Bending to the side (i.e., lateral flexion).

3. **Rotation:** Twisting and turning.

It is helpful to know these three planes of movement. However, we rarely move in just one plane when dancing (we usually move in a combination of two, or all three, planes).

24. Spine Like a Slinky
(Rounding and Arching the Spine)

Purpose: To find both connection and differentiation between the individual vertebra of the spine for more even distribution of effort and increased mobility from pelvis to head.

Where Used: A great warm-up for shaping, backbends, body rolls and general dancing. Also, for Follower's frame in Smooth and Standard (as the upper spine is extended).

Position: Sitting.

1. Sitting in a chair, begin to gently round your back. Return to neutral and repeat several times. As you round, allow your head to look down and the top of your pelvis to move backward (i.e., flattening the curve in your lower back). Become aware of how you do this movement—this is far more valuable than achieving a large range of motion.

2. Look toward the ceiling and gently arch your spine. Return to neutral and repeat several times. As you arch, allow your belly and top of your pelvis to move forward.

3. Smoothly combine steps 1-2, rounding and arching your whole spine. In your mind's eye, watch the changing curve of your spine. Find how to distribute the effort from pelvis to head, imagining each vertebra moving an equal amount.

4. Pick a point in front of you. Keeping your eyes looking at that point, begin to gently round and arch your spine (the movement will be smaller than before). Allow your head to move while your eyes look forward—when your head lowers, you look out the top of your eyes; when your head is lifted, you look out the bottom of your eyes. After a few repetitions, return to letting your head move with the rest of your spine.

5. (Optional): Return to step 3 and notice your breathing. Are you inhaling or exhaling when you round your spine? Continue this pattern of breathing a couple more times, and then do the opposite (e.g., if you were exhaling while arching, change to inhaling while arching and exhale when rounding). Do this a few times, and then return to breathing in whatever way feels most comfortable to you.

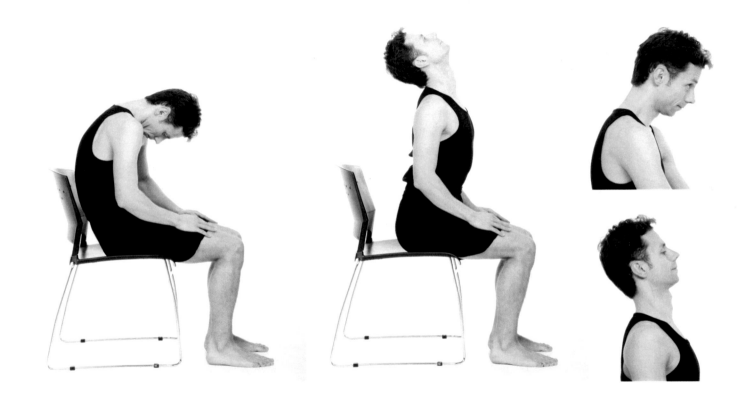

25. Grow Two Inches Taller

(Lengthening the Spine)

Purpose: A quick way to improve posture.

Where Used: A great preparation for dancing.

Position: Standing.

1. Imagine there is a large helium balloon tied to the crown of your head. Rise onto your toes as high as possible (i.e., onto the platform), growing taller and taller. Imagine that the balloon helps lift you from the top of your head.

2. Without getting any shorter, slowly lower your heels back to the floor. Of course this is impossible, but it is a great way to lengthen the spine.

3. Repeat steps 1-2 a couple more times.

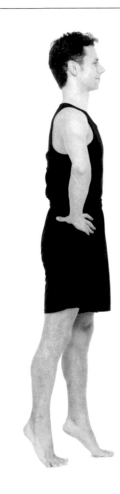

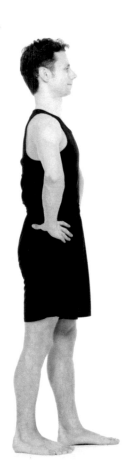

26. Tallest/Shortest Mountain

(Bending the Legs and Maintaining Upper Body Alignment)

Purpose: To be able to change elevation without affecting the verticality of the spine or position of the pelvis.

Where Used: Whenever rising, lowering or bouncing.

Position: Standing against a wall and then walking.

1. Stand with your back toward a wall, with your heels and sacrum touching the wall. Think of lengthening your spine, minimizing (but not eliminating) the curves of your lower back and neck. Bring as much of your back (as is comfortable) into contact with the wall. Lengthen the back of your neck and gently bring your head to meet the wall (or come as close to the wall as is possible for you right now).

2. Feel the whole backside of your torso and head supported in the vertical by the wall. Slowly walk away from the wall, retaining this feeling of length, width and support.

3. Return to standing with your back against the wall. Bend your knees, allowing your back to slide down the wall. Then slowly straighten your knees, sliding your back up the wall. Sense when your knees are fully straight but not locked. Repeat this several times, paying attention to your upper body alignment. Lower only as far as you are able to without changing the alignment of your pelvis or spine. Use the wall for feedback.

4. Come away from the wall. Stand with upright posture and imagine yourself as a tall mountain. Bend and straighten your knees as you did before, this time maintaining your alignment without the wall. As you bend your knees, notice if the torso part of your mountain gets shorter. It should remain long and in the same alignment.

5. Standing as the tallest mountain (with knees straight), take five steps forward, getting slightly lower on each step. As the shortest mountain (i.e., on the fifth step), have you maintained your upper body posture?

6. From this lowered position, take five steps forward. Get slightly higher on each step, so that you finish at your tall-mountain height. Repeat steps 6-7 a few times.

7. Repeat steps 6-7 walking backward.

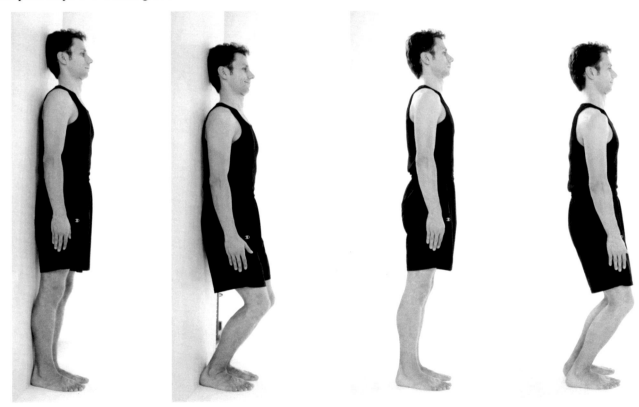

Top Pointers for the Spine

1. Lengthen your spine without eliminating the curves of your back (*Grow Two Inches Taller*).

2. Keep your spine aligned, yet flexible (i.e., do not stiffen your spine) (*Spine Like a Slinky*).

3. Remember that it is possible to move the other joints in your body while maintaining the alignment of your spine (*Tallest/Shortest Mountain*).

4. *Move* your whole spine together when moving through space (rather than leaning).

5. Generally speaking, turning your spine will turn your whole body.

Chapter 7
Head and Neck

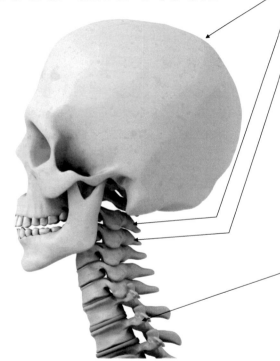

Bones and Joints of the Head and Neck

Skull: Bony structure of the head and face.

Atlas: First cervical vertebrae. The atlas is the very top of our spine upon which the skull rests.

Axis: Second cervical vertebrae. The axis forms the pivot upon which the atlas and head rotate.

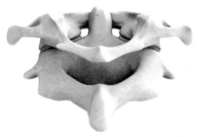

Atlas and Axis *(rear view)*

Seventh Cervical Vertebra: The large bottom vertebra of the neck.

Functions of the Head and Neck

Most of our senses are located in our head—eyes, ears, nose, mouth and inner ear (sense of balance). Humans are highly visual—our eyes scan the environment, look in the direction we want to move, and generally leads the way for the rest of our body. Therefore, our head is primary to our movement and balance. While the neck is, of course, part of the spine, we are including it in this chapter due to its key role in moving the head.

By having more awareness, we are able to increase the freedom of motion of our head and neck, improve our posture and alignment, establish better balance and more!

27. Get to Know Your Head and Neck

Locate various bones of your head and neck:

- **Skull:** Feel the whole circumference of your skull. You might even feel your lower jaw and how it hinges from your skull.

- **Atlas:** It is not particularly easy to feel with the hands. Instead, place your fingers at the openings of your ears—this is approximately the level at which your skull rests on your atlas vertebra. Nod your head "yes" to help feel this place.

- **Axis:** It is not easy to feel with the hands. Instead, turn your head "no" to help feel this vertebra just below the atlas.

- **Seventh Cervical:** Find the large, knobby vertebra at the base of the neck. This is your seventh cervical, commonly called C7.

28. Knuckle Biter

(Minimizing the Curve of the Neck)

Purpose: To feel the muscles that lengthen the back of the neck and bring the head into better alignment.

Where Used: Everywhere.

Position: Standing and walking.

1. Make your right hand into a fist and gently bite onto your index finger (your right elbow is lifted and out to the side).

2. Lengthen the back of your neck while gently resisting with your index finger. You move your neck slightly backward while pulling your finger slightly forward. Feel how this minimizes the curve at the back of your neck and brings your head into a balanced alignment.

3. Repeat steps 1-2 using your left hand.

4. Biting the index finger of your choice, begin to walk around the room with the finger and neck gently resisting each other.

5. Lower your hand and walk around the room, maintaining the newfound length in the back of your neck.

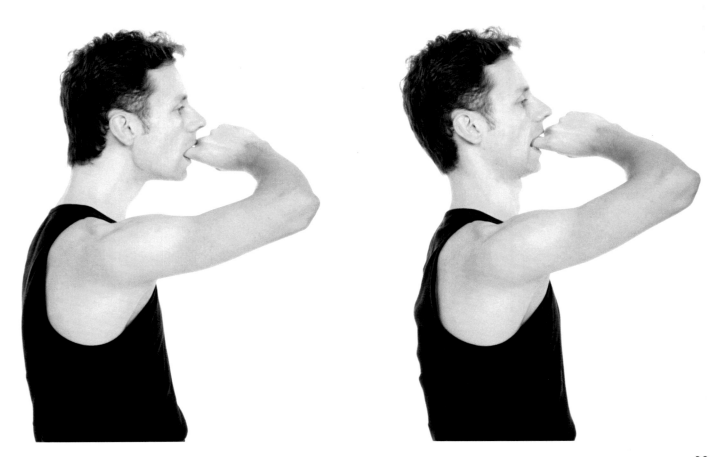

29. Block Head

(Aligning the Head)

Purpose: To increase awareness of the whole circumference of the head in order to improve head alignment.

Where Used: In all of Rhythm and Latin, and for the Leader in Tango.

Position: Standing and walking.

1. Imagine your head as a square block. Arrange the block of your head so that the top and bottom are parallel to the floor.

2. Lengthen your head toward the ceiling, thinking of lifting the entire block from the center of its top. Make sure to keep the block parallel to the floor. Find the horizon with your eyes.

3. Begin to walk around the room, maintaining this lifted and parallel alignment of the block of your head. Experiment with turning your head and walking backward as well.

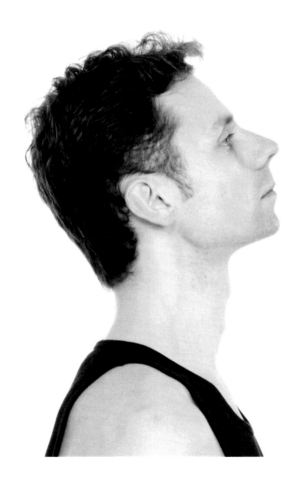
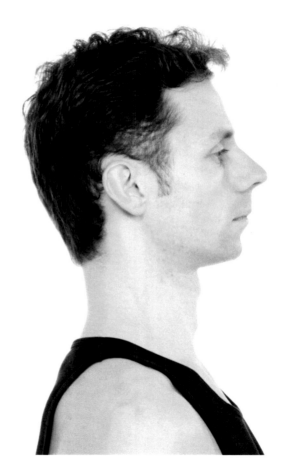

30. Paint the Ceiling

(Moving the Spine in One Piece)

Purpose: To move the spine in one piece for better balance, efficient movement and complete weight shifts. Also great for improving alignment of the head and neck.

Where Used: On every step (except when purposefully doing otherwise).

Position: Sitting.

1. Sit at the front of a chair. Take a moment to feel how you are sitting on your sit bones.

2. Imagine your spine is the stick or handle of a large paint brush. The stick starts at your sacrum, continues up through the column of your neck and out the crown of your head. On the very top of this stick is the brush.

3. Imagine that the ceiling lowers to be right above your head. Begin to paint a forward and back line on the ceiling. Since your head and spine are like a stick, they move together in one piece (i.e., you will need to bend in your hip joints). Brush over this line many times.

4. Paint a line right and left (i.e., perpendicular to the one you just painted). Brush over this line many times.

5. Paint a circle several times in one direction, and then the other. direction.

6. For contrast, imagine that the stick of the paint brush starts at the base of your neck. Begin to paint a few circles with just your head and neck (the rest of your spine is now quiet). Notice how this is different than moving your head from your sacrum. Then return to moving the whole spine in one piece.

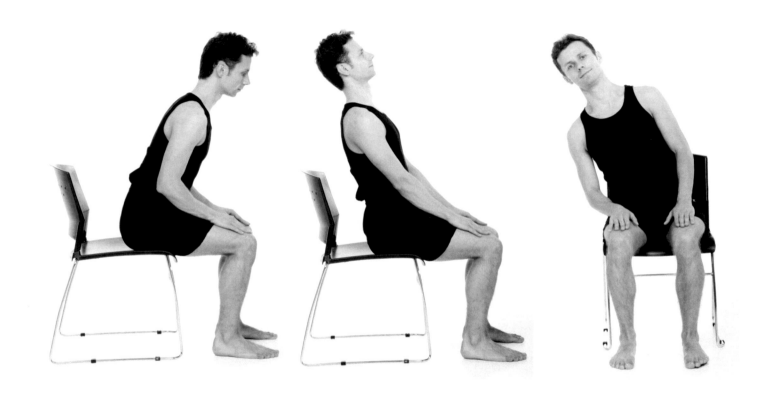

31. Just Say No

(Turning the Head from the Axis)

Purpose: To discover how to turn the head from the highest place possible—the axis (second cervical vertebra). This lengthens the neck and reduces effort, creating clean lines.

Where used: Whenever changing the direction of your face (e.g., turning to Promenade Position, spotting during turns, snapping the head for dramatic styling, etc.)

Position: Sitting or standing.

1. Sitting or standing, get a sense of where your atlas and axis vertebrae are (see *27. Get to Know Your Head and Neck*).

2. Think of initiating your axis vertebra, begin to slowly turn your head right and left. Think that your neck lengthens and your head is almost floating on the top of your spine. While the other vertebrae in your neck will also turn, focus on smoothly rotating your axis around your atlas—the very top vertebra of your spine.

3. For contrast, simply turn your head right and left without thinking about the axis or lengthening your neck. Compare the quality and range of turning. Then return to initiating the turn from your axis vertebra.

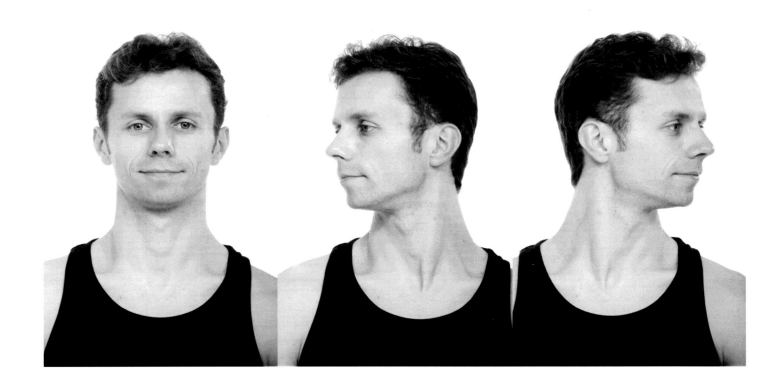

32. Jewel of the Spine

(Connecting the Movement of the Spine and Head)

Purpose: To feel the connection of the head to the rest of the spine for organic movement and alignment, especially during shaping and sway.

Where Used: Whenever you change weight, sway or shape.

Position: Standing.

1. Stand tall, lengthening your spine. Notice where your head rests on top of your spine (i.e., base of the skull and atlas vertebra). Gently nod your head "yes" to help feel this place.

2. Think of your head as a jewel that is an extension of your spine. Imagine there is light shining up out of the jewel (i.e., out the crown of your head).

3. Begin to shift weight side to side, taking a small left foot side step (brushing the right foot closed to the left foot) and then a small right foot side step (brushing the left foot closed to the right foot). Imagine your spine and jewel as a stick that moves in one piece as you shift weight.

4. Now, step side on the left foot but keep the right toes on the spot so that the right leg is extended to the side. With weight on the left foot, tilt your jewel-spine stick to the left to create a diagonal line from the right toes to the top of the jewel.

5. Repeat step 4 stepping the right foot side and tilting right.

6. Imagine your jewel-spine is now a flexible stick, like a young tree branch that bends in the wind. Begin shifting weight side to side, swaying your spine (i.e., as weight shifts onto the left foot, the jewel and spine sway right, and as weight shifts onto the right foot, they sway left). Focus on flowing the movement and curve of the spine through the neck and into the jewel so that the head is truly an extension of the spine.

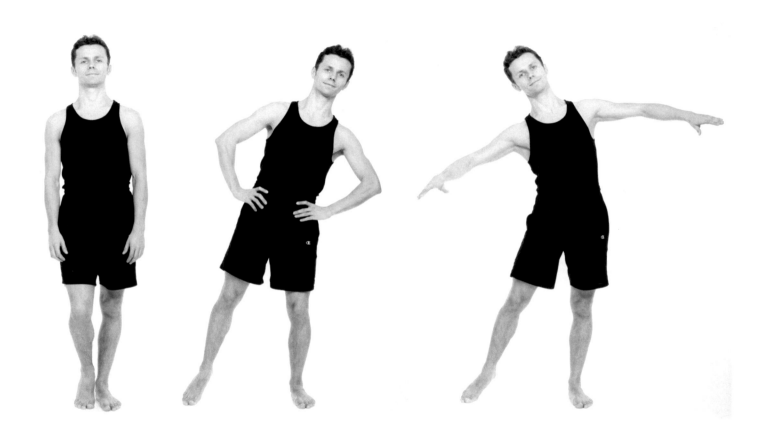

Top Pointers for the Neck and Head

1. Remember that your neck is part of your spine and your head is its jewel. Allow your head and neck to respond to the alignment and movement of your spine (*Paint the Ceiling* and *Jewel of the Spine*).

2. When lengthening your head upward, think of lifting the top of your head (i.e., do not tilt your head back) (*Block Head*).

3. In the Rhythm and Latin dances, keep the block of your head parallel to the floor, especially when turning (*Block Head*).

4. For more refined turning of your head, think of turning from the axis (i.e., second) vertebra (*Just Say No*).

5. Pay attention to where your eyes look. This has tremendous influence on how you move your head and neck (and the rest of yourself).

Chapter 8
Rib Cage

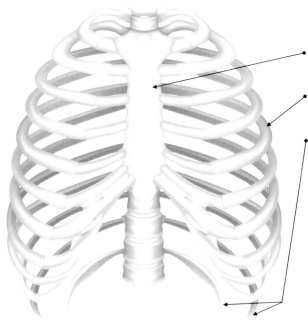

Bones the Rib Cage

Rib Cage: The bony and cartilaginous structure of the chest, also called the *thoracic cage*. The rib cage is comprised of the ribs, sternum, and the cartilage that connects them (with the exception of the floating ribs).

Sternum: The long flat bone at the front of the chest. Also called the *breast bone*.

Rib: An individual long curved bone of the rib cage. We have 12 pairs of ribs—10 of which connect with the sternum.

Floating Ribs: The lowest 2 pairs of ribs, shorter than the rest. The floating ribs do not connect with the sternum, making them particularly flexible.

Diaphragm: The thin, dome-like muscle that extends across the bottom of the rib cage and is the primary muscle of breathing (not pictured).

Functions of the Rib Cage

The main functions of the rib cage are to protect our vital organs and help in respiration (i.e., breathing). The diaphragm attaches to the inner circumference of the bottom of the rib cage, separating our chest and abdominal cavities. The diaphragm is responsible for approximately 75% of our respiration—the collective movement of the ribs accounts for the rest.

The ribs connect with the vertebra in back, intimately linking their movement with that of the spine. Each rib slopes downward as it wraps from back to front, and then attaches to the sternum directly (ribs 1-7), indirectly through costal cartilage (ribs 8-10) or not at all (ribs 11 and 12). The rib cage also widens from top to bottom—the lower ribs are about three times as wide as the first rib.

Despite the name rib *cage*, the ribs are very flexible, able to expand, contract and even move separately from each other (to a small degree). Being more aware of our ribs and sternum improves our alignment and expands our ability to twist, sway and shape.

33. Get to Know Your Rib Cage

In sitting or standing, locate the bones of your rib cage:

- **Rib Cage:** Feel the whole circumference of your rib cage. Include touching where the ribs join the sternum in front, where the ribs meet your spine in back, and the ribs under your arm pits. You might also follow one rib along part of its length, noticing how it slopes downward from back to front.

- **Floating Ribs:** Find the bottom of the front your rib cage. Gently running your fingers a little up and down, follow along the bottom edge of the rib cage toward your sides. You will find your first pair of floating ribs before you reach your sides. If you continue, you may be able to feel your other pair of floating ribs, which end approximately at your sides.

- **Sternum (Breast Bone):** Find the notch at the front base of your neck. Feel from this top part of your sternum, down to where it ends at the solar plexus.

34. Accordion Ribs

(Opening and Closing the Sides of the Ribs)

Purpose: To increase awareness and flexibility of the ribs and thoracic spine.

Where Used: Swaying and shaping in all dances, as well as using the ribs in Latin hip action.

Position: Sitting.

1. Sit on a chair. Lightly place the palm of your right hand on the top of your head, with your right elbow to the side. Use your hand to slowly bend your head to the right (as if to bring your right ear to the shoulder). Return to neutral and repeat several times. Keep your face forward (i.e., do not turn your head).

2. Lift the right side of your pelvis a small amount. Feel how your weight shifts to the left side of your pelvis. Lower and repeat a few times. Notice what happens in the ribs on your right side and left side.

3. Place your right hand on top of your head again. Gently bend your head to the right while lifting the right side of your pelvis. Feel how your whole right side folds while the left side opens, similar to the bellows of an accordion. Return to neutral and repeat several times. Find how to distribute the effort more and more evenly through your whole spine.

4. Repeat steps 1-3 on the other side (i.e., using your left hand, bending to the left).

5. Interlace both hands and place them on the top of your head. Begin to alternately bend your head and arms to the right and left. Go slowly and notice which side is easier. When done, lower your hands.

6. Alternately lift the right and left sides of your pelvis, keeping your head in the middle (you may interlace your hands on top of your head to check that it is staying vertical). Observe how your ribs and spine bend underneath your head.

7. Interlace your hands on top of your head. Begin to bend your head to the right while lifting the right side of your pelvis. Return to neutral. Then bend your head to the left while lifting the left side of your pelvis. As you continue alternating right and left several times, sense the changing shape of your spine and ribs.

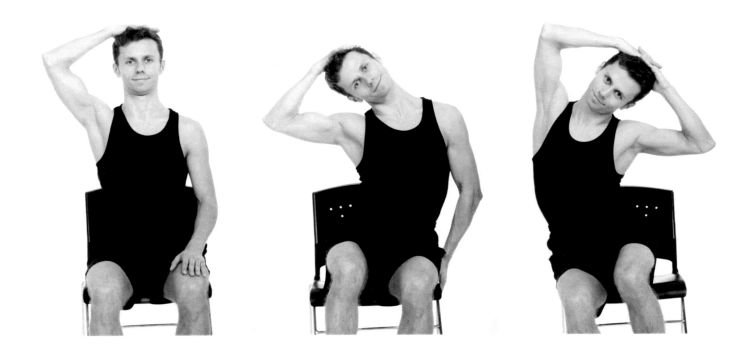

35. Blowfish

(Breathing into the Back and Sides of the Ribs)

Purpose: To include the backs and sides of the rib cage in breathing, for more width and stability when dancing.

Where Used: Everywhere.

Position: Standing or sitting.

1. Stand or sit on a chair. Without changing anything, simply observe your breathing. Which parts of you move as you inhale? Do you breathe more into the belly or chest? Do you sense movement at the sides or back of your ribs?

2. Begin this pattern of breathing: inhale, expanding your chest and then exhale, expanding your lower abdomen (do not arch your back). Imagine you are a blowfish that is alternately puffing up the chest and the abdomen. Repeat this a few times.

3. Using the same breathing pattern, this time completely exhale all the air while expanding your lower abdomen. Hold your breath for a few seconds and then exhale a little more air (if comfortable, do this another time or two). Then wait until you spontaneously inhale.

4. Take a few normal breaths and then repeat step 3.

5. Breathe normally and notice what has changed from the beginning. Do you sense more movement in the sides and backs of your ribs as you inhale?

6. Now place your hands on your lower ribs at your sides and in back (i.e., right above your waist), with your fingers pointed backward and thumb forward. Feel the movement of your breathing there. Use your hands as a way to invite air into this area, allowing your ribs to expand into your hands.

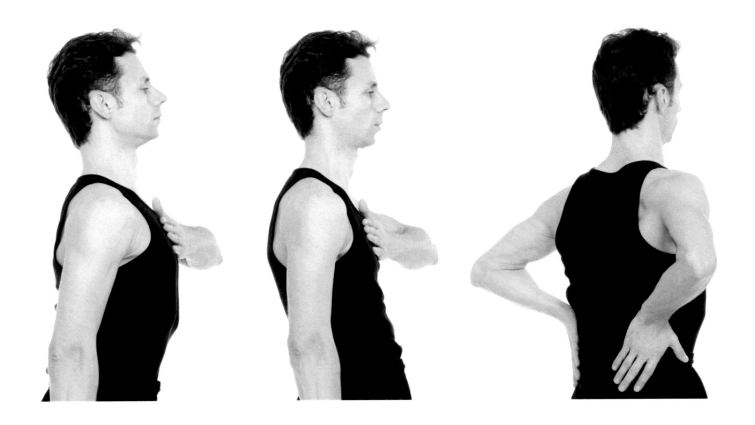

36. Light Beam

(Aligning the Rib Cage and Sternum)

Purpose: To include the sternum in your awareness for improved rib alignment and presentation.

Where Used: Everywhere.

Position: Sitting with back against a wall, then standing.

1. Sit on the floor against a wall. At first, touch only your upper back to the wall. Then move your lower ribs back to meet the wall. This serves to place the rib cage in a good alignment (i.e., the front lower ribs are closed while the ribs in back are wide). Feel the whole length of your back supported by the wall.

2. Slowly come to standing. Find this same alignment of the rib cage, and then walk around, maintaining this alignment without being stiff.

3. Stand and imagine placing a small light in your belly button. Walk around the room, letting this light lead the way—that is, allow your lower ribs and abdomen to protrude and move ahead of the rest of you. This is an exaggerated version of the common mistake of letting the lower ribs pop out.

4. In your imagination, move the light to the top of your sternum, where the clavicles and first rib meet the sternum. Walk around, projecting this beam of light and thinking that it leads the rest of you. Use this helpful image when dancing to keep your back long and your ribs aligned. Make sure that the beam is attached to your sternum (not pushed ahead of your body), so that you do not get top heavy.

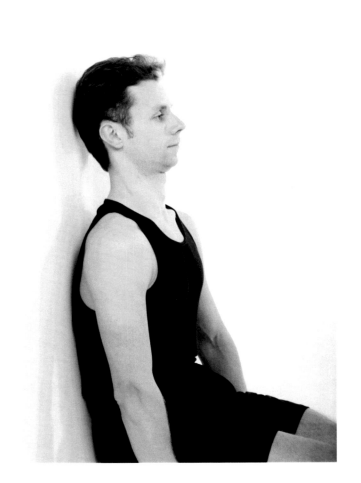
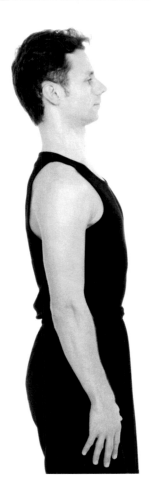

37. Lace Up Your Corset

(Closing the Lower Ribs)

Purpose: To learn how to close the lower ribs to establish good alignment of the rib cage.

Where Used: Everywhere.

Position: Standing.

1. In standing, imagine that you have two popsicle sticks lying flat against the front of your ribs—one on the right side and one on the left.

2. Experiment and find how to tilt the bottoms of the popsicle sticks forward or backward by changing the alignment of your rib cage. Gradually find the alignment of the rib cage that allows the popsicle sticks to be completely vertical.

3. Now imagine that the popsicle sticks are the boning of a corset you are wearing. This corset is sturdy yet elastic. Place your hands on your lower ribs in front and imagine your fingers are the laces of the corset.

4. As you exhale, gently lace up the corset by bringing your hands toward each other and a little inward toward the spine. Feel the sensation of the lower ribs closing in front. Tie the laces and enjoy the support of the imaginary corset in maintaining the alignment of your ribs.

5. With your hands still on your lower ribs, observe the movement of your breath. Notice that you can still breathe (including into the back of the rib cage) easily since the corset has some stretch. However, while the lower ribs expand and contract with the breath, the alignment of the rib cage is not disturbed (i.e., the lower ribs do not pop out in front as you inhale).

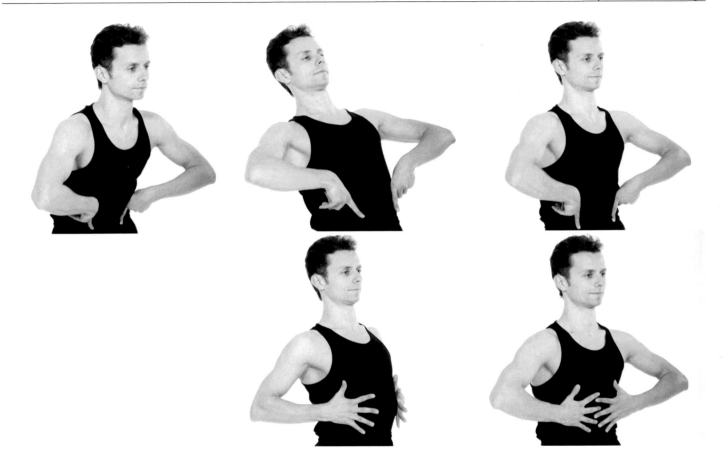

38. Build a Spare Room

(Creating Space Between the Ribs and Pelvis)

Purpose: To lengthen the ribs away from the pelvis for improved posture, mobility and stability.

Where Used: Everywhere.

Position: Standing and walking.

1. Stand normally and notice the distance between the bottom of your rib cage and the top of your pelvis (i.e., your waist area). You might use your hands to feel this distance.

2. Imagine there are several heavy weights hanging around the circumference of the bottom of your rib cage. Let the weights sink your ribs lower and lower, as if the block of your rib cage is in an elevator going down to the floor below (i.e., your pelvis). Observe that the space between your ribs and pelvis decreases or even disappears. Walk around and see what this posture feels like.

3. Imagine the weights are removed and your rib cage takes the elevator up to the third floor. Sense the space between your pelvis and rib cage getting longer and feel your bellybutton moving closer to your spine. This is your spare room, now on the second floor. Walk around and see how this compares to when your ribs were sitting in your pelvis. As you walk, imagine your building is vertical and sleek without any balconies jutting out (i.e., your ribs are smoothly aligned with your waist and pelvis).

4. Observe the connection between the pelvis and rib cage made by the spare room. Feel the strength and stability of your waist area held by the framing of your spare room.

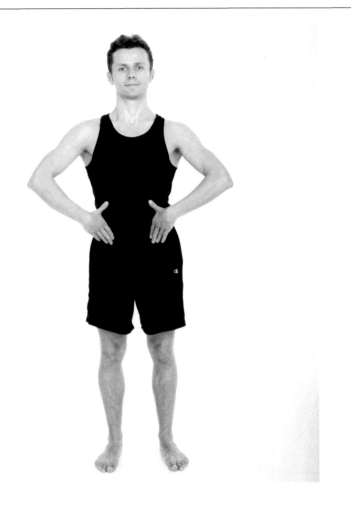
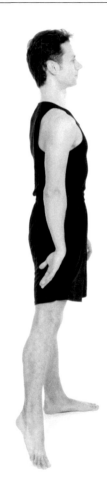

Top Pointers for the Rib Cage

1. Maintain a neutral alignment of your rib cage (*Lace Up Your Corset*).

2. Think of closing your floating ribs in front, without any force or holding your breath (*Lace Up Your Corset*).

3. Lift the block of your rib cage away from your pelvis (*Build a Spare Room*).

4. Connect your rib cage and pelvis with imaginary elastic girdle for support and stability (*Build a Spare Room*).

5. Shine the light of your sternum, moving it through space as you dance (*Light Beam*).

6. When creating sway, make sure not to collapse the other side of the rib cage.

7. Breathe in all three dimensions—forward, side and back. Bringing your breath toward the back of your lungs helps creates width and stability (*Blowfish*).

Chapter 9
Shoulder Girdle

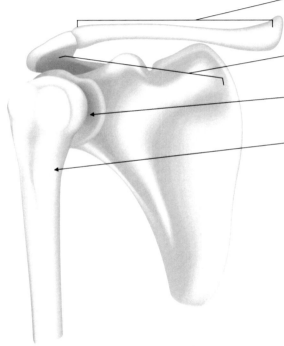

Bones and Joints of the Shoulder Girdle

Clavicle: The long horizontal bone at the front of the upper chest, also known as the *collar bone*. Each clavicle runs from the sternum to its shoulder joint.

Scapula: The flat, triangular-shaped bone that sits on the upper back of the rib cage, also called the *shoulder blade*.

Shoulder Joint: The place where the upper arm meets the torso (i.e., the glenohumeral joint between the scapula and humerus).

Humerus: The bone of the upper arm.

Functions of the Shoulder Girdle

The two main functions of the shoulder girdle are to give the arms and hands a tremendous range of motion and the strength and stability to use them to lift, push, pull, etc.

The shoulder is similar to the hip joint in that both allow a large degree of freedom of movement. However, the shoulder is more complex, involving three joints (as opposed to just one in the hip joint). There is the joint where the upper arm bone articulates with the scapula (glenohumeral joint). A second joint involved in movement of the shoulder is between the scapula and the clavicle (i.e., the acromioclavicular joint). The third joint is the only point at which the arm connects to the central part of our skeleton—where the clavicle meets the sternum (i.e., the sternoclavicular joint). In short, the upper arm connects to the scapula, the scapula connects to the clavicle, and the clavicle connects to the sternum.

Being aware of how our shoulder girdle works allows for greater ease and range of motion in our arms and chest, increases the effectiveness of our frame and partner connection, improves the quality of our posture and helps create a clean top line.

39. Get to Know Your Shoulder Girdle

In sitting or standing, locate the bones and joints of your shoulder girdle:

- **Clavicle (Collar Bone):** Starting at the top of your sternum, find where your clavicles connect (i.e., the sternoclavicular joint). Thus follow the length of each clavicle out to its shoulder.

- **Scapula (Shoulder Blade):** Reach your hand over the opposite shoulder to find the shoulder blade. The easiest landmark to feel is the bony ridge near the top of the shoulder blade.

- **Shoulder Joint:** Find where the outer edge of the scapula and the upper arm bone come together. This is your shoulder joint.

- **Partner Exercise:** Standing behind a partner, place each of your hands on his or her shoulder blades. Slowly trace the outline of one of your partner's shoulder blades and then the other, giving your partner a clear sense of their shape, size and location. Make sure to find the bottom tip of each shoulder blade. Switch roles and repeat.

40. Shimmy Shoulders

(Exploring Movements of the Shoulders)

Purpose: To increase awareness of how the shoulders move to enable smoother and more coordinated movement and to improve frame and presentation.

Where Used: Shimmies, Spanish drag, styling, etc.

Position: Sitting.

1. Sitting on a chair, gently raise your right shoulder toward your ear. Slowly return to neutral and then lower your shoulder a small amount toward the floor. Return to neutral and repeat several times, allowing your right arm to simply hang. Notice how your right shoulder blade and clavicle also move. Place your left hand on your right clavicle to clarify how it moves.

2. Repeat step 1 with your left shoulder. Notice any differences from your right shoulder.

3. Begin to move your right shoulder (including the clavicle and shoulder blade) a little forward and back. Keep your rib cage and spine quiet, so that your shoulder moves independently (i.e., do not turn your chest with your shoulder). Feel how your shoulder blade slides away from your spine (when the shoulder moves forward) and toward your spine (when the shoulder moves back). Observe how your clavicle hinges from the joint at which it connects to the sternum. Place your left hand on your clavicle to better feel its movement.

4. Repeat step 3 with your left shoulder. Compare any differences you find between your left and right shoulders.

5. Begin to slowly circle your right shoulder forward (i.e., up, forward, down and back) several times. Focus on the quality and smoothness of the circle, *not* the size. Change directions, circling your shoulder backward several times.

6. Repeat step 5 with your left shoulder. Are the circles with this shoulder smoother or more bumpy?

7. Move both shoulders forward, as if they wanted to touch in front. Then move both shoulders back, as if to touch each other behind. Repeat this several times while keeping your chest, spine and head more or less still. Feel the independent movement of your shoulder girdle. In particular, notice the movement happening at the joints between your clavicles and sternum (i.e., the sternoclavicular joints).

8. Move the right shoulder forward while taking the left shoulder back, and then switch—moving the left shoulder forward while taking the right shoulder back. This is similar to how the shoulders move in walking (i.e., natural contrabody movement). Gradually decrease the size of your movements while increasing the speed, so your shoulders begin to shimmy.

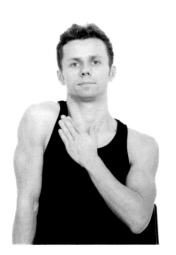 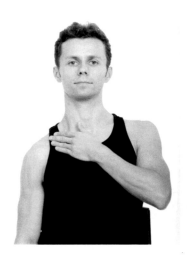 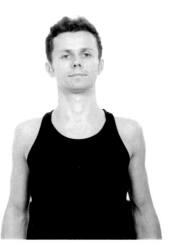 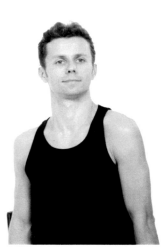

41. Anchors Away

(Rolling the Shoulder Blades Down)

Purpose: To position the shoulder blades so as to improve frame, partner connection and top line, and to create width and stability.

Where Used: Everywhere.

Position: Standing with a partner.

1. In pairs, have a partner stand behind you and place his or her palms on your shoulder blades. Throughout this exercise, your partner will softly assist the movement of your shoulder blades with his or her palms.

2. Gently slide your shoulder blades up toward your ears. Then slide them down toward your waist (without power).

3. Together with your partner, slide your shoulder blades away from your spine (i.e., spreading them wide toward the sides of the ribcage). Then slide your shoulder blades toward your spine (i.e., bringing them closer to each other).

4. Switch roles with your partner and repeat steps 2-3.

5. Again, have your partner stand behind you and place his or her palms on your shoulder blades. Anchoring the shoulder blades uses two of the four directions you have explored—*down* and *away* from the spine. Together with your partner, move your shoulder blades down and away from the spine.

6. Complete the anchoring of your shoulder blades by tipping the bottom point of each shoulder blade toward the front of the body (i.e., inward, toward the ribs). Have your partner gently press the points of your shoulder blades down and forward using the heels of his or her hands. Sense the corresponding feeling in your chest of slightly lifting and opening.

7. Ask your partner to slowly release the hands while you maintain the anchored position of your shoulder blades.

8. Switch roles with your partner and repeat steps 5-7.

Having experienced anchored shoulder blades, you can re-establish them without repeating this whole exercise. *I Dream of Jeannie* (next exercise) and *Turning Doorknobs* (Chapter 10) are also good exercises to anchor your shoulder blades.

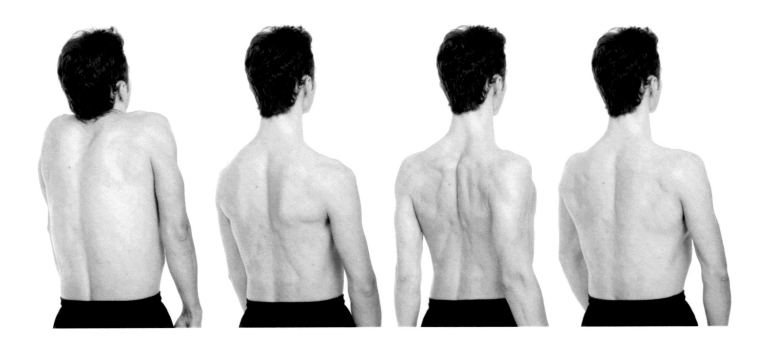

42. I Dream of Jeannie

(Broadening and Anchoring the Shoulders)

Purpose: To widen and anchor your shoulder, in order to give strength to the upper body and improve presentation.

Where Used: Everywhere, especially in dance frames and creating Promenade Position.

Position: Sitting (or standing).

Note: The name of this exercise was inspired by a 1960's American television show in which Jeannie uses her magical powers by folding her arms (in the position used in this exercise) and blinking her eyes.

1. Sitting on a chair, extend both arms forward at about shoulder height. Bend your arms and take hold of the opposite elbow with each hand. Your forearms are crossed, with one wrist above and one below. Your palms cup your elbows, and your thumbs and fingers are closed together.

2. Pretend that your arms are a drawer. Gently slide this drawer a little out and in (i.e., away from and in toward your chest). As the drawer slides out, your forearms move away from your chest and your shoulders are pulled forward. As the drawer slides in, your forearms come closer to your chest and your shoulders move back. End with the drawer in (i.e., shoulders back).

3. Begin to widen your shoulders and elbows out to the sides, while keeping your shoulders and shoulder blades down. Resist slightly with your hands so that your arms do not break apart from each other. Feel how your shoulder blades slide away from the spine and your back widens.

4. Switch your arms (so that the wrist previously on top is now below) and repeat steps 2 and 3.

5. With your arms crossed either way, slowly lengthen your right elbow forward and return to neutral. Do the same with your left elbow. Continue to alternately lengthen each elbow and upper arm. Keep your head and rib cage still while allowing your shoulder joints to move. Feel how the lengthening arm's shoulder blade widens even further on your back, and the outside end of the clavicle travels forward.

6. Having established broad, anchored shoulders, slowly release your hands from your elbows and position your arms into a Closed Position frame (as either Leader or Follower).

7. Change the shape of your frame to Promenade. Do this by slightly lengthening the upper arm (left for Leaders and right for Followers) and allowing that shoulder blade to move away from the spine. Then return your frame to Closed Position. Repeat transitioning between Closed and Promenade Positions several times.

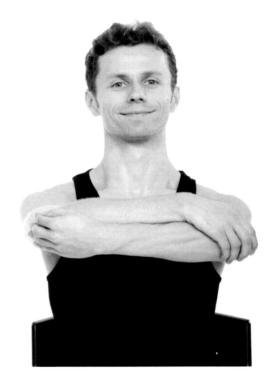

Useful Image: Another quick way to experience broad, anchored shoulders is to imagine that you are wearing a well starched shirt. Sense where the press line would be along the outside of each sleeve. Then imagine that someone gently pulls each press line out to the side, widening your elbows and shoulders.

43. SeeSaw Shoulder

(Using the Shoulder Blade as a Counterweight to the Arm)

Purpose: To coordinate the movement of the shoulder blade in response to raising the arm, so that the shoulder stays down.

Where Used: Every time an arm is raised to or above shoulder height, including taking a frame with a partner.

Position: Standing or sitting.

1. Standing, extend your right arm out to the side at shoulder height. Begin to raise your right arm up, taking your shoulder with it (i.e., hiking your shoulder up toward your ear). This is a common mistake. Return your arm to shoulder height.

2. Imagine your right arm and shoulder blade are like a seesaw (i.e., teeter-totter)—your right hand and shoulder blade are the two ends and the pivot point (i.e., fulcrum) is your shoulder joint (i.e., where your humerus meets your shoulder blade). Unlike a playground seesaw, your seesaw is uneven (i.e., the pivot point is much closer to one end).

3. Imagine a child sits on the shoulder blade end of your seesaw, causing your right arm to raise up. Then imagine another child sits on the hand end of your seesaw, causing your arm to lower again. Continue playing with this movement. Become clearer about the seesaw relationship between your arm and shoulder blade—when your arm raises, your shoulder blade lowers and its bottom tip rotates more to your right side. Also, observe that your clavicle remains fairly quiet and horizontal throughout the entire movement.

4. Repeat steps 1-3 with your left arm.

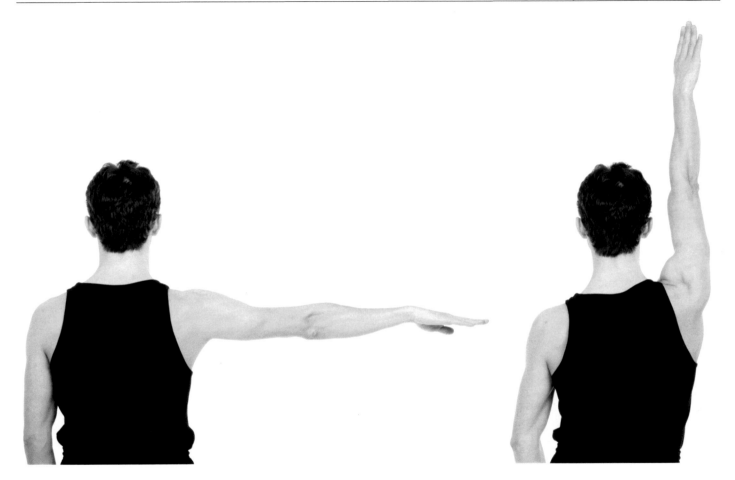

44. Wringing the Towel

(Rolling the Collar Bones and Arms in Opposition)

Purpose: To clarify the relationship between the collarbones, arms and spine, as well as to coordinate use of the arms with the torso (e.g., hip and rib action).

Where Used: Arm styling in dances with rhythmic body action (i.e., Rhythm and Latin).

Position: Standing.

1. Stand and extend your arms to your sides at shoulder height with your palms facing down. Make soft fists with your hands.

2. Begin to rotate each fist clockwise (i.e., the inside of your right wrist starts turning toward the front while the left starts turning toward the back). Return to neutral and repeat several times. Feel the connection of both arms through your clavicles. You might imagine that your fists are the two ends of a wet towel that you are wringing out.

3. Rotate each fist counter clockwise (i.e., the inside of the left wrist now starts turning toward the front and the right turns to the back). Return to neutral and repeat a few times.

4. Combine the movements of steps 2 and 3, turning both fists one direction, returning through neutral and then rolling in the other direction. You may want to do it a few times with your hands open and see how it affects the movement. Then add turning your head to look toward the hand turning upward.

5. Return to the movement of step 4. Add lengthening the arm of the hand turning upward. Allow the arm to pull your ribs, upper spine and other arm along. Do not make a large movement— simply become aware of the coordination happening between the bones and joints of your arms, chest, spine and head. Repeat several times.

6. Return to the movement of step 5, this time turning your head toward the hand turning down and back. Do this several times, paying attention to how it is different. Then again, turn your head toward the hand turning upward.

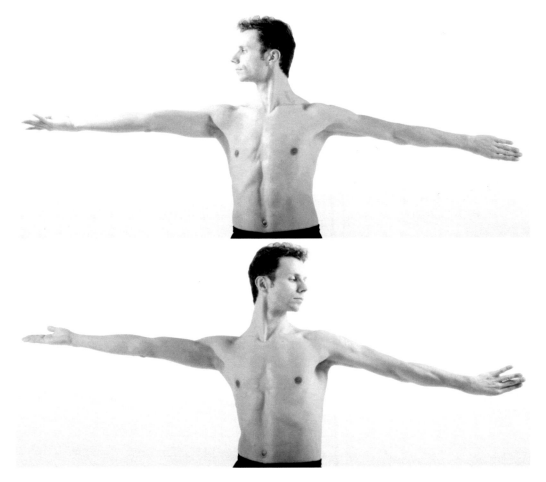

Top Pointers for the Shoulder Girdle

1. Anchor your shoulder blades down and away from your spine (*Anchors Away*). This does not mean your shoulder blades are fixed—allow them to slide as necessary.

2. Keep your shoulders wide and down without forcing them down (*I Dream of Jeannie*).

3. Open your chest so that your clavicles are wide, with a feeling of being rolled up and back (*Anchors Away,* and *Turning Doorknobs* in the next chapter).

4. Allow your clavicles to participate in your movement—especially the movement of your arms and chest (*Wring the Towel*).

5. Whenever your raise your arm, allow your shoulder blade to slide down and out—but only as far as needed to counterbalance the movement of the arm (*SeeSaw Shoulder*).

Chapter 10
Arms and Hands

Bones and Joints of the Arms and Hands

Humerus: The bone of the upper arm.

Elbow Joint: The joint between the upper and lower arm comprised of all three bones (humerus, ulna and radius). The elbow is primarily a hinge joint that allows the arm to bend and straighten.

Ulna: One of the two long bones of the forearm, on the little finger side.

Radius: The other long bone of the forearm, on the thumb side.

Wrist Joint: Where the radius bone articulates with the first row of carpals.

Phalanges: The bones of the fingers. There are two phalanges in the thumb and three in each of the fingers.

Metacarpals: The five long bones between the wrist and fingers.

Carpals: The eight small bones of the wrist.

Functions of the Arms and Hands

Our arms and hands are vital to our lives (e.g., eating, bathing, reaching, lifting, etc.). The ability to bend at the elbows allows us to change the distance between our shoulders and hands, and the elbow and wrist joints allow us to turn our forearms to have are palms up (supination) or down (pronation).

Our hands, with their opposable thumbs, are a unique aspect of being human and have a large range of mobility. They are also highly versatile, capable of making fine, delicate movements, as well as transmitting power from our center.

Understanding more about how the arms and hands move results in improvements in leading and following skills, your frame, and arm and hand styling.

45. Get to Know Your Arms and Hands

Locate the bones and joints of your arms and hands:

- **Humerus (Upper Arm Bone):** Gently squeeze along your upper arm, feeling for the bone underneath the muscles. Now bend your arm and find the round bony parts on either side of the point of your elbow—this is the lower end of your humerus.

- **Ulna:** Feel this bone on the little finger side of your forearm. Its lower end is the bony knob just above your wrist. Its upper end is the point of your elbow.

- **Radius:** Turn your palm up and feel this bone running along the thumb side of your forearm. When the palm is up like this, the ulna and radius are parallel to each other. Now, slowly turn your palm to face down. See if you can feel the radius crossing the ulna.

- **Elbow Joint:** Place a hand on the outside of the opposite elbow. Bend and straighten the elbow, feeling how the three bones (humerus, ulna and radius) articulate with each other.

- **Wrist Joint:** Gently run your fingers over the top of your wrist to feel the eight small bones of the wrist. Then hold the lower ends of your radius and ulna (the knobs on either side of your wrist). Bend and move your wrist to feel the joint in action.

- **Metacarpals (Hand Bones):** Feel the five metacarpals that connect to your fingers through both the top and palm of your hand.

- **Phalanges (Fingers):** Touch your fingers, noticing that the thumbs have only one knuckle while the other fingers have two.

46. Turn on the Hose
(Visualizing the Lines of the Arms)

Purpose: To clarify the connection between the arms and spine for refined quality in arm movement and positioning, and partner connection.

Where Used: In all frames and arm styling.

Position: Standing or sitting.

1. Stand or sit on a chair with your arms resting at your sides. Imagine a line running down through the inside of your right arm and out the end of your middle finger. Follow this line from the right shoulder joint through your upper arm, elbow, forearm, hand and middle finger.

2. Then extend the line of your right arm from your shoulder to your seventh cervical vertebra (the bump at the base of your neck in back). Think that your arm actually begins at this point on your spine. In your mind's eye, trace the entire line (from spine to finger) several times, clarifying any parts that are unclear.

3. Now imagine this line is a garden hose. Turn on the water at the base of your neck. Feel the water flow through the length of the hose and shoot out the end of your middle finger.

4. Keeping the hose and water in your awareness, begin to move your right arm through various positions used in dancing (i.e., out to the side, above the head, forward, etc.).

5. For comparison, rest your right arm and begin to move your left arm. Do you feel a difference in quality from your right arm?

6. Repeat steps 1-4 with your left arm.

7. Finally, do steps 3 and 4 with both arms.

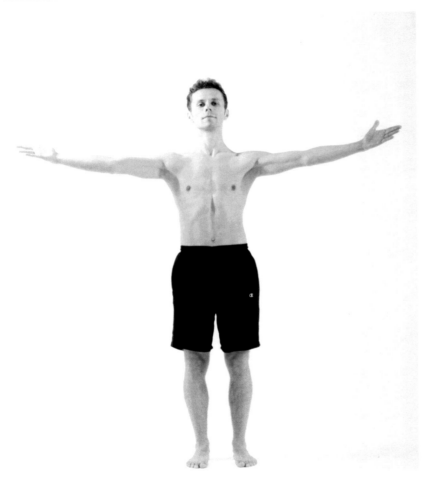
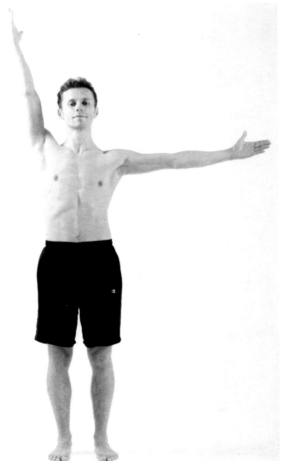

47. Turning Doorknobs

(Turning the Upper and Lower Arm Together and Separately)

Purpose: To become aware of how the upper and lower arms move together or separately when extended to the sides or overhead. This expands and refines the possibilities for arm styling, shaping and frames.

Where Used: In all arm styling, shaping and frames.

Position: Standing or sitting.

1. Stand or sit on a chair. Extend both arms sides and slightly forward at shoulder height. Have your palms facing forward.

2. Imagine each hand is holding a doorknob. Turn these imaginary doorknobs forward by turning just your forearms and wrists (i.e., your palms turn in the direction of the floor). Return to neutral and repeat a few times. Observe how your elbow joints act like pivot points, allowing your forearms to rotate while your upper arms remain quiet.

3. Turn the doorknobs forward again, but this time let your upper arms turn as well (i.e., your entire arms are now turning in their shoulder joints). Return to neutral and repeat. Notice how your shoulder blades move upward as your arms turn forward.

4. From the original starting position, begin to turn the doorknobs backward. Turn only your forearms and wrists (i.e., your palms turn in the direction of the ceiling). Return to neutral and repeat a few times. Then allow your upper arms to turn as well. Observe how your shoulder blades move down.

5. Using your whole arms, turn the doorknobs forward and then backward. Do this slowly, staying within a comfortable range. Notice what the quality of your movement is like. Does one arm/shoulder move more easily?

6. Begin moving your head and shoulders with your arms. As you turn the doorknobs forward, gently look down and let your upper back round. Then as you turn them backward, look up, allowing your sternum and upper chest

to lift. As you repeat this, pay attention to what your collar bones and shoulder blades are doing.

7. Return to turning the doorknobs using only your arms. What is the quality and range of your movement like now?

8. One last time, turn the doorknobs backward. Leaving your upper arms as they are, turn just your forearms forward until your palms face downward. Sense how the energy of your arms remains up and out. This is the feeling you want to have when dancing and when connecting with a partner. This is last step is also a great shortcut to anchoring your shoulder blades (as in *Anchors Away*).

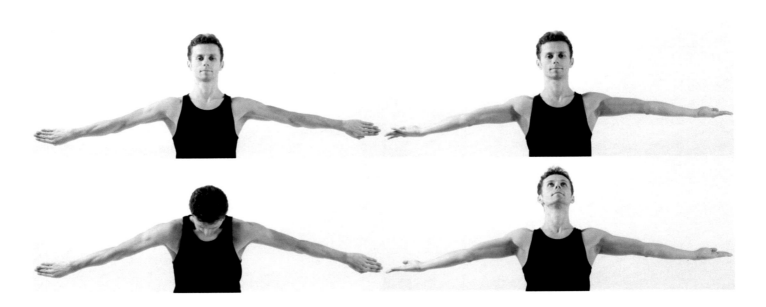

48. Go Bowling

(External Rotation of Upper Arm)

Purpose: To create an upward energy in open position frames for a light, positive partner connection.

Where Used: All single and double handhold connections.

Position: Standing.

For Followers

1. Standing, imagine you are holding a lightweight bowling ball in your right hand. With your palm facing forward, move your arm backward in preparation for throwing the bowling ball. Then swing your arm forward, releasing the imaginary ball. Notice that your arm ends in a lifted and externally rotated position.

2. Throw the bowling ball again and leave your right arm in the air. Keeping your upper arm externally rotated, gently turn your palm downward (your forearm also turns). Maintaining the shape of your arm, lower your right hand and place it into your imaginary Leader's hand. Feel how the external rotation of your upper arm gives your arm a light, upward energy. Repeat this a few times.

3. For contrast, let your right arm hang at your side. Without thinking about it, simply place your right hand in your imaginary Leader's hand. What is the energy of your arm like now?

4. Repeat steps 1-3 with your left arm.

For Leaders

1. Standing, imagine you are holding a lightweight bowling ball in your left hand. With your palm facing forward, move your arm backward in preparation for throwing the bowling ball. Then swing your arm forward, releasing the imaginary ball. Notice that your arm ends in a lifted and externally rotated position.

2. Throw the bowling ball again and leave your left arm in the air. Keeping your upper arm externally rotated, gently turn your palm to face rightward (your forearm also turns). Maintaining the shape of your arm, lower your left hand and offer it to your imaginary Follower. Feel how the external rotation of your upper arm gives your arm a light yet connected energy. Repeat this a few times.

3. For contrast, let your left arm hang at your side. Without thinking about it, simply offer your left hand to your imaginary Follower. What is the energy of your arm like now?

4. Repeat steps 1-3 with your right arm.

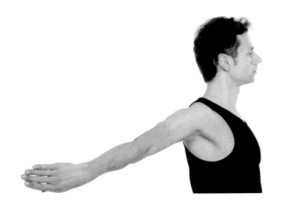
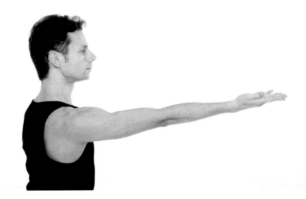

49. Hand Wave

(Turning the Hands In and Out)

Purpose: To position the hands in a way that maintains openness of the front of the torso.

Where Used: In all dance frames, including open positions.

Position: Sitting.

1. Sit on a chair and bend your left arm so the forearm is parallel to the floor. Turn your palm down and spread your fingers wide. Imagine you are wearing a form-fitting long-sleeve shirt with two seams—one that run alongs the inside edge of your forearm and another the runs along the outside edge. Notice the angles at which the thumb and little finger sides of your left hand flare out from the lines of your shirt's seams.

2. Move your left hand to the left (from the wrist) until your thumb is in line with the inner seam—that is, forming a straight line from the inside of your elbow to the tip of your thumb. It is as if your hand is "turned out." Then do the opposite—move your left hand to the right until your little finger is in line with the outer seam. It is as if your hand is "turned in." Alternate between these two positions a few times.

3. "Turn out" your left hand (with palm out and thumb up) so there is a straight line from your inner forearm to the end of your thumb. Keeping your hand turned out, begin to extend your left arm in the direction of your middle finger (i.e., diagonally leftward). Notice how the left side of your chest widens.

4. "Turn in" your left hand (with palm out and thumb down) so there is a straight line from your outer forearm to the end of your little finger. Keeping your hand turned in, let your middle finger lead the arm rightward, to fold in and close to your chest.

5. Repeat steps 1-4 with your right hand.

6. Repeat steps 3-4 using both arms simultaneously. Observe how the angle between your wrists and hands effects your arms, shoulders and chest.

7. Take a partner in a Closed Position frame. Turn out your hands and notice the feeling in your frame. Then turn in your hands and feel how it is different. Again, return to turning out your hands.

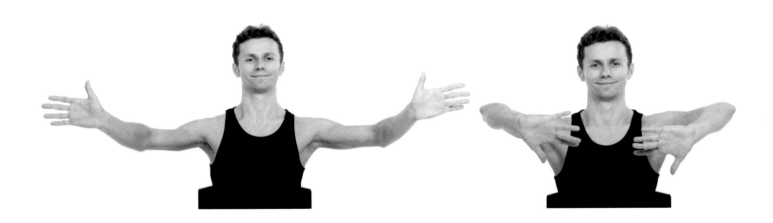

50. Grow a Glove Size

(Spreading the Bones of the Hands)

Purpose: To discover how much movement is possible in the hands for better articulated hand styling.

Where Used: Hand styling.

Position: Sitting.

1. Sitting on a chair, make "jazz hands" with both hands (i.e., spread your thumbs and fingers). Look at your hands, taking note of their shape.

2. Gently spread and massage the bones of your right hand (i.e., the metacarpals) with your left hand. Then take hold of the end of your right little finger. Gently lengthen the finger and begin to turn the finger around its axis. Feel not only the bones of the finger but the metacarpal as well. Imagine the muscles softening to give the bones complete freedom of movement.

3. Repeat step 2 with each of other fingers and the thumb of your right hand.

4. Sense the five metacarpal bones of your right hand. Make a "jazz hand" with your right hand thinking of spreading these bones. See and feel the difference from before.

5. Repeat steps 1-4 with your left hand.

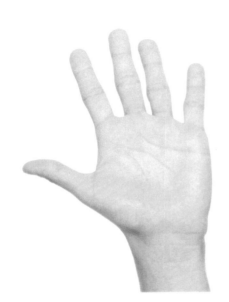
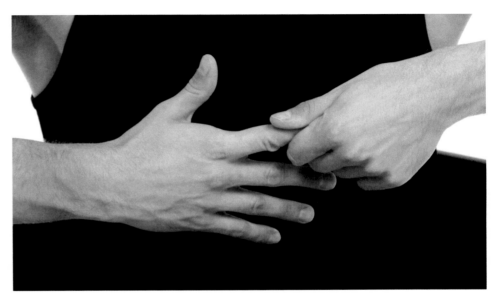

51. Magic Hands
(Circling the Wrists and Fingers)

Purpose: To differentiate the fingers and improve the coordination between them, as well as the wrist, for more precise and beautiful hand styling.

Where Used: Hand styling.

Position: Sitting.

1. Sitting on a chair, slowly circle your right wrist in one direction. After several times, circle in the other direction.

2. Begin to make circles again, this time leading with your right middle finger. After several times, circle in the other direction.

3. Practice Follower's hand styling by spreading the fingers of your right hand. Then, starting with your little finger, slowly circle each finger clockwise in succession from your wrist. Do this several times, finding a smooth coordination of your wrist and fingers.

4. Practice Leader's hand styling by closing the thumb and fingers of your right hand. Circle your hand and fingers from your wrist, keeping the thumb and fingers closed.

5. Repeat steps 1-4 with your left hand. For steps 3-4, circle counter clockwise (instead of clockwise).

6. For a fun challenge, circle both hands at the same time, either as Follower or Leader. Magic!

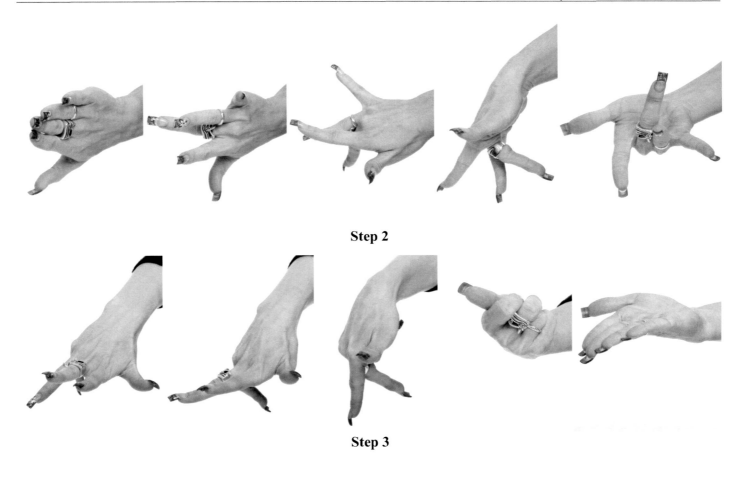

Step 2

Step 3

52. Pray for a Good Frame

(Connecting the Arms to the Torso)

Purpose: To cultivate the ability to move the frame from the torso for better leading and following.

Where Used: All frames, especially when turning.

Position: Standing.

1. Stand comfortably. Place your hands in a prayer position against your sternum (i.e., the middle of your chest).

2. Begin to turn your chest and shoulders a little left and right (i.e., twisting your spine) while keeping your head facing forward. Notice how your arms simply go along for the ride. Continue until you have a clear sense of how your arms move together with your torso.

3. Shape your arms into a Closed Position frame (as either Leader or Follower). Begin to twist your spine a little left and right while keeping your head facing forward. Retain the same feeling as when your hands were against your chest. Are you able to keep your arms connected to and moving with your torso?

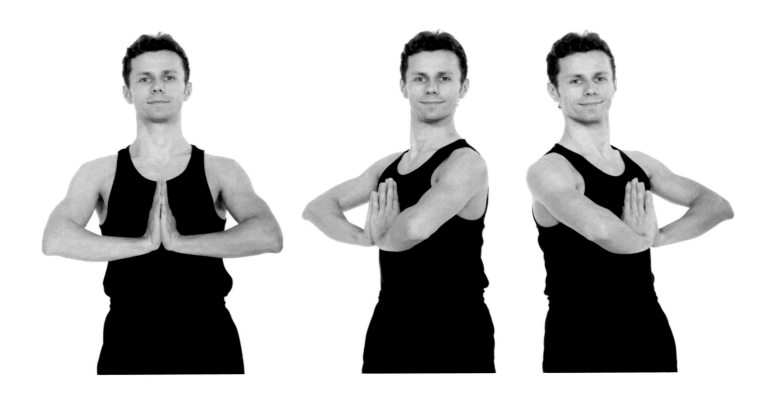

53. Parallelogram

(Positioning the Arms in a Smooth and Standard Frame)

Purpose: To find the position of the arms in relation to the torso that allows for effective leading in a Closed Position Smooth and Standard frame.

Where Used: Closed Position Smooth and Standard frame.

Position: Standing.

1. Stand tall and bend your right arm into a Leader's Closed Position Smooth or Standard frame.

2. Keeping your elbow bent, move your right upper arm forward and back in the shoulder joint to get a sense of its range of motion. Imagine a pane of glass parallel to the front of your body that is touching the front of your right hip bone (i.e., the ASIS). Move your right elbow to also touch the pane of glass, so that your elbow and hip bone are in line with each other (i.e., your right elbow is slightly in front of the body).

3. Tie an imaginary string from your right hand to your right knee. Begin to twist right and left on your feet, taking the rest of yourself along. Keep the imaginary string taut, and your hand and knee in the same vertical line (i.e., your right hand cannot go past your midline).

4. Relax your right arm at your side and arrange your left arm into a Leader's Closed Position frame. Explore the forward and back range of motion of your upper left arm in the shoulder joint. Gradually position your arm so that your left elbow is in line with your left shoulder joint (i.e., the elbow is in the same line as the shoulder joint).

5. Arrange both arms into a Leader's Closed Position frame. Position your right elbow and hand as in steps 2-3, and your left elbow as in step 4. Notice that your two arms are not equally forward—the right elbow is more forward than the left. Take a moment to feel the shape of this frame.

Note: The Follower's parallelogram is like the Leader's—the left upper arm extends directly side, and the right hand clasps the Leader's left hand (so the Follower's right elbow is in front of the right hip bone).

Parallelogram with a Partner

1. Take a partner in Closed Position. As Leader, start with both elbows extended directly in line with your shoulder joints (i.e., neither forward nor back). The shape of your frame is square.

2. As the Leader, move your right elbow forward to be in line with the front of your right hip bone (leave your left elbow in line with its shoulder). The Follower's left elbow is in line with the left shoulder and the right hand joins with the Leader's left hand (which means the Follower's right elbow is more forward than the left). Observe how, together with your Follower, the shape of your frame is like a parallelogram.

3. For contrast, try the opposite parallelogram by first returning the frame to being square (as in step 1). Then, as the Leader, move your left elbow forward, in line with your left hip bone (keep your right elbow in line with its shoulder). Notice how this opposite parallelogram feels. Return to the original parallelogram (step 2). Which of the two parallelograms is the most comfortable?

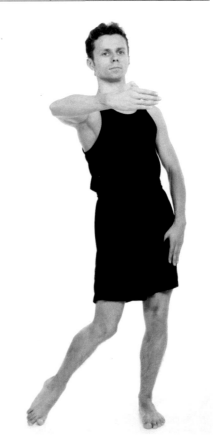

54. Release the Butterflies

(Creating Upward Energy in the Arms)

Purpose: To create an upward energy in the arms for a light, positive partner connection, increased elegance and better balance.

Where Used: Closed frames and when addressing an audience.

Position: Standing.

1. Standing tall, lift your arms in front of you at shoulder height.

2. Imagine there are beautiful butterflies in your belly. Sense these butterflies as they travel up your spine and fly through the length of both arms. Imagine releasing these butterflies from the middle of each palm. Allow the light movement of the butterflies to create an upward energy in your arms as you expand them into a Closed Position frame. You may also imagine butterflies flying out of your upper chest.

3. Take a partner in Closed Position. Think of releasing the butterflies. Notice how light, yet connected, this feels.

4. For contrast, forget about the butterflies and allow your frame to lose some of its upward energy. Observe what this does to the partner connection. Then return to using the butterflies to create an upward energy in your frame.

Correct

Incorrect

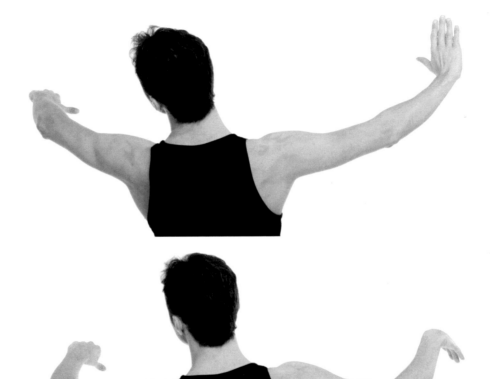

Top Pointers for the Arms and Hands

1. Think of lengthening your upper arms away from your torso, creating space in your shoulder joints.

2. Even when your arms are straight, allow your elbows to be slightly soft, not locked.

3. Make sure your arms do not fall behind the plane of your shoulders.

4. Keep your upper arms slightly externally rotated (*Turning Doorknobs*). This anchors the shoulder blades, establishes a positive partner connection, and creates a nice neck and shoulder line (*Anchors Away* from the previous chapter).

5. When connecting with a partner, maintain an upward energy in your arms (*Go Bowling* and *Release the Butterflies*) and an openness in the front of the torso (*Hand Wave*).

6. When raising your arm (e.g., for an underarm turn), think of lifting from your elbow rather than the hand.

7. When an arm is free (i.e., not touching your partner), keep it alive and an active extension of your movement by sending energy from your center, through your arms to your fingertips (*Turn on the Hose*).

8. Be intentional in how you move your arms—do not leave it to chance.

Chapter 11

Whole Body Integration

This book has divided the body into separate sections for learning purposes. However, we are not a compilation of parts—we are one person. Since everything is connected, a change in one aspect of ourselves has ripple effects on the rest of ourselves. As we become more aware of these connections, we gain greater mastery over our movement.

Whole body integration cultivates our ability to pay attention to one part of ourselves without losing sight of the rest. For example, when practicing Latin hip action, we must focus on the details of how our femurs and pelvis move while also maintaining a global awareness of what is happening elsewhere, in our neck and spine, feet, breathing, etc.

Looking in a mirror to see, and using our hands to feel, how we move are both valuable means of feedback. It is also essential to cultivate our internal kinesthetic awareness. Practicing tuning into the proprioceptive messages from our joints, muscles and other bodily sensations develops this to be an immediately accessible and accurate source of feedback that is always available to us. Be curious to discover the details you feel when doing a movement or dancing a figure. Is there a place where the movement stops or gets disturbed? How can the movement flow smoothly through your entire skeleton?

In dancing, it is often said that posture is everything. It is true that good posture is the key to reliable balance, powerful movement, solid partner connection and a professional appearance. The main regions of a dancer's body are often referred to as "blocks of weight" (i.e., the head, shoulders, ribcage and pelvis). When our blocks of weight are stacked up appropriately, we are said to have good posture. However, since we are continually moving when dancing, good posture is really good dynamic alignment (i.e., being poised to move in any direction at any moment). Dynamic alignment includes both the ability to stack up our blocks of weight on every step, as well as to consciously choose to move a part of ourselves separately (i.e., body isolations).

55. Stack Up the Blocks

(Aligning the Blocks of Weight)

Purpose: To find a balanced alignment of the body's main blocks of weight (head, shoulder, rib cage and pelvis) over the feet.

Where Used: Everywhere.

Position: Standing.

1. Stand tall with balanced alignment. Move the block of your head forward a small amount, taking it slightly out of alignment. Sense how this changes your balance and overall alignment, then return your head to neutral. Next, move your head a little backward, taking it out of alignment to the back. Return to neutral. Repeat the same thing to the right and to the left, observing how it effects your balance. Finally, take a moment to feel the block of your head in its neutral alignment. Is your neutral place more clear now?

2. Repeat step 1 with the block of your shoulders (i.e., move the shoulders out of alignment to the front, back, right and left).

3. Repeat step 1 with the block of your ribs, then your pelvis.

4. Standing with all of your blocks of weight in alignment, shift the weight on your feet forward toward the balls of the feet. Return to neutral. Repeat the same thing to the back (i.e., toward your heels), to the right (i.e., to the outside of your right foot and inside of your left foot), and to the left. Return to a neutral place of the weight on your feet.

5. Stand with your blocks in alignment and the weight in a neutral place on your feet. Take a step forward on one foot and re-establish a balanced alignment. Then take a step on the other foot and do the same.

6. Repeat step 6, taking backward steps.

7. Optional Variations: Take a step and turn to the left or right, flex your knees, or create a shape, re-establishing a balanced alignment.

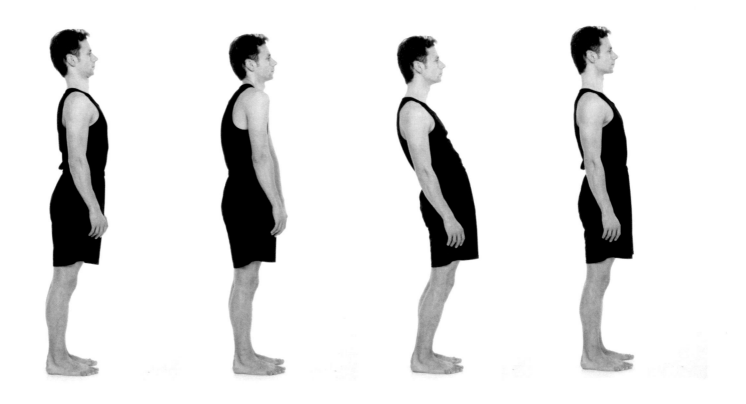

56. Rubik's Cube
(Differentiate and Coordinate the Head, Shoulders and Pelvis)

Purpose: To improve flexibility and coordination of the head, shoulders and pelvis to turn separately or together in various combinations.

Where Used: Anytime the head, shoulders or pelvis need to turn separately from or in combination with each other. Examples include promenade position, grapevines and Latin hip action.

Position: Standing.

1. Stand square to a wall in a comfortable stance. Remember where you are standing, as you will return to this spot.

2. Slowly turn to your right (as if to look at something over your right shoulder). Return to neutral and repeat a few times. Notice how far you see comfortably without stretching. Remember the place that you see for comparison later.

3. Turn a small amount to the right (i.e., less than half of your capability). Keeping your shoulders and hips where they are, begin to turn only your head a little right and left. Think of scanning the horizon with your eyes. Then, begin to move your eyes opposite to your head (i.e., as your head turns right, your eyes look to the left and vice versa). Allow your breathing to be easy and your jaw to be soft. Return everything to neutral and walk a few steps to refresh yourself. Then repeat step 2.

4. Turn a small amount to the right. Keeping your head and pelvis still, turn only your shoulders a little right and left several times. Then, slowly turn your head in the opposite direction of your shoulders (your pelvis remains still). Return everything to neutral, walk a few steps, and then repeat step 2.

5. Turn a small amount to the right. Keeping your head and shoulders still, turn your pelvis a little right and left several times Then, add turning your shoulders opposite to your pelvis, (your head remains still). Optional: After a few times, begin to turn your head in the same direction as your pelvis while the shoulders turn opposite (i.e., your head and pelvis turn right as your shoulders turn left and vice versa). Return everything to neutral, walk a few steps, and then repeat step 2.

Note: You may repeat the exercise turning to the left. However it is not necessary, as you will automatically integrate the learning and transfer it to the other side.

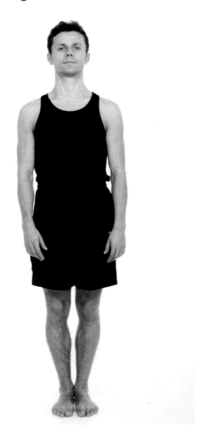
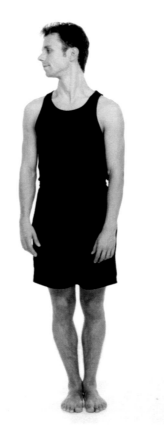
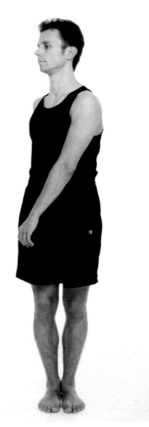

57. Give Yourself Goosebumps

(Moving the Joints When Dancing)

Purpose: To discover the importance and pleasure of moving the joints when dancing.

Where Used: Everywhere!

Position: Standing.

1. Play an upbeat song that makes you want to dance.

2. On your own, begin to freestyle dance as you wish (i.e., without any prescribed movements). Think of dancing your bones and joints. Bend and turn as many joints as possible, moving your bones through space. Have fun—play with making silly shapes, gesturing with the arms, bending lower to the floor, traveling, etc.

3. Continue dancing, moving as little as possible in your joints. Notice how this feels.

4. Return to moving in as many joints as possible. Notice how much more satisfying this feels. You might even give yourself goosebumps!

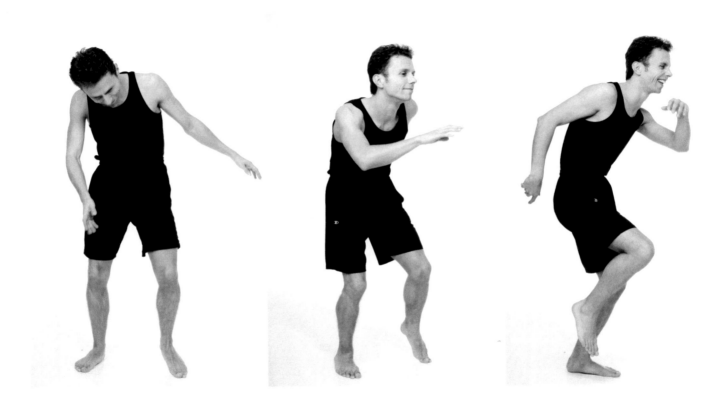

58. A Leg to Stand On

(Standing on One Leg)

Purpose: To improve balance and dynamic alignment for smooth, controlled transfer of weight from foot to foot.

Where Used: Every step.

Position: Standing.

1. Stand comfortably. Step side on your right foot and pick your left foot off the floor. Find the alignment that allows you to balance easily standing on the right leg. Then step side on your left foot and do the same thing. Continue this several times.

2. Repeat step 1 taking forward steps, then taking back steps.

3. Repeat step 1, taking steps in all four directions (mixing them in various ways).

4. Repeat steps 1-3, brushing your free foot closed to the standing foot (instead of picking up your free foot).

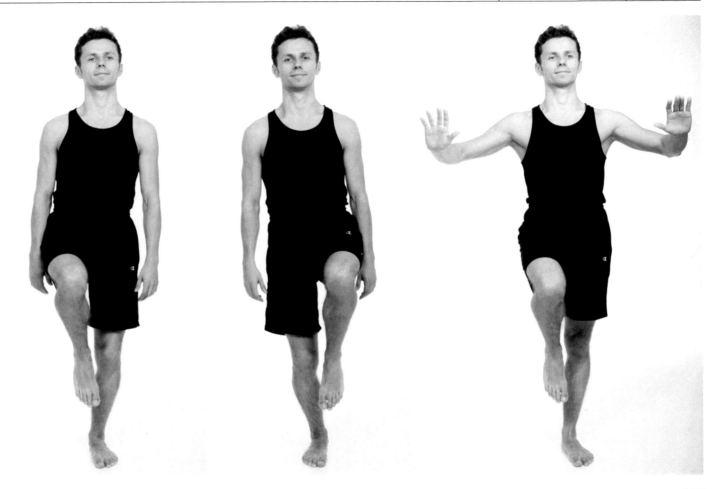

59. Balance is Good Medicine

(Playing Toss Standing on One Leg)

Purpose: To develop better balance by challenging stability and dynamic alignment.

Where Used: Every step.

Position: Standing.

Prop: Medicine ball or other ball with some weight to it.

1. With your ball, stand about 8-10 feet from your partner. Stand on your left leg with your right foot lifted from the floor.

2. Toss the ball back and forth with your partner while remaining on one leg.

3. Repeat step 2 standing on your right leg (with your left foot lifted).

4. If you want more challenge, vary the trajectory, height and speed at which you and your partner throw the ball. If the ball is small enough, experiment with catching it with one hand.

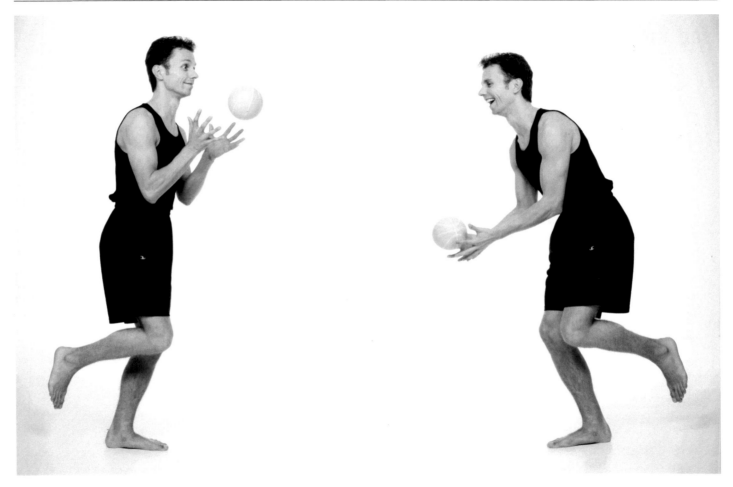

Top Pointers for Whole Body Integration

1. Stand as tall as possible, with a feeling of the energy being "up" (*Grow Two Inches Taller*).

2. Maintain balanced, dynamic alignment of all your blocks of weight (head, shoulders, rib cage and pelvis). This will allow you to move easily in any direction (*Stack Up the Blocks*).

3. If you move a block of weight out of alignment, have it be a conscious choice (*Stack Up the Blocks*).

4. Reduce any unnecessary muscular effort so that you are truly dancing on your bones (*Put a Spring in Your Step*).

5. Allow your breathing to be free and continuous.

Chapter 12
Dynamic Alignment While Moving

Moving from foot to foot is a continuous process of giving up and recovering our stability. In this dynamic process, we are perpetually aligning ourselves for balance. Even when standing still we are moving—our bones, joints and muscles continually make small adjustments to stay upright in gravity. These internal organizations are also essential for preparing us to take a step, create a shape and connect with a partner when dancing.

Generally, the more our blocks of weight are in alignment and move together, the more powerful and smooth our weight shifts and walks will be. Refining the initiation of movement and weight transfer will dramatically improve the quality of your dancing.

60. Going Without Going

(Weight Shifting on One Foot)

Purpose: To cultivate internal movement *before* stepping for smooth weight transfer to the next step, as well as a richer overall quality of dancing.

Where Used: Before every step.

Position: Standing.

1. Stand with weight on your right leg. Begin to shift your weight forward and back on your right foot several times. Feel the movement in your ankle, as well as how your femur moves forward and back.

2. Shift your weight a little right and left (i.e., toward the outside and inside edges of your right foot) several times. Then take a few steps around to refresh yourself.

3. Again standing on your right leg, shift your weight in a circle on your foot, connecting the four points—front, right, back and left. Track the circular movement in your ankle. Notice if your right femur is also moving in a circle. After a few times, change the direction of the circles.

4. Repeat steps 1-3 standing on your left leg.

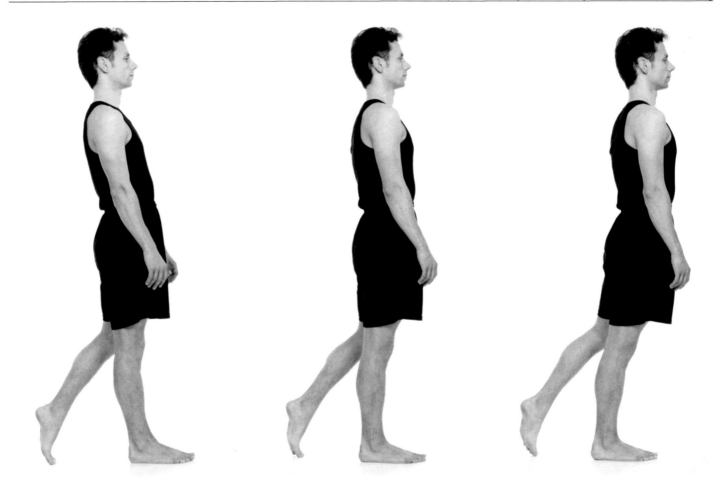

61. Put on Your PJs

(Preparing to Step in the Smooth and Standard Dances)

Purpose: To put the *Move Like a Champion*® principles to use when preparing to step in Smooth and Standard.

Where Used: In preparation for all steps in Tango, and stepping forward or back on count 1 in the other Smooth and Standard dances.

Position: Standing.

Smooth and Standard Dances (Other than Tango)

1. Stand on your right leg with your blocks of weight lined up.

2. "P" is for Pounds: Really sense that your blocks of weight (pounds) are over your right leg.

3. "J" is for Joints: Simultaneous with sensing your pounds, pay attention to the joints used in lowering: the hip, knee, and ankle. Bend these joints in coordination and lower on your right leg (as in *Smooth Operator*).

4. "S" is for Spine: With your pounds aligned and joints flexed, take a left foot forward step, moving your entire spine in one piece (as in *Paint the Ceiling*).

5. Repeat steps 2-4 a few times from standing on your right leg, and then from standing on your left leg.

6. Repeat steps 2-4 stepping backward (do each leg).

Tango: So far, you have lowered from your standing height, as you would on count 1 in most Smooth and Standard dances. However, in Tango, your standing knee will already be flexed.

1. Stand on your right leg with the knee slightly flexed. Repeat Pounds-Joints-Spine, noting that you lower less than in the previous exercise. After a few times, start standing on your left leg.

2. Repeat step 1 stepping backward (do on each leg). Then repeat step 1 stepping to the side (do on each leg).

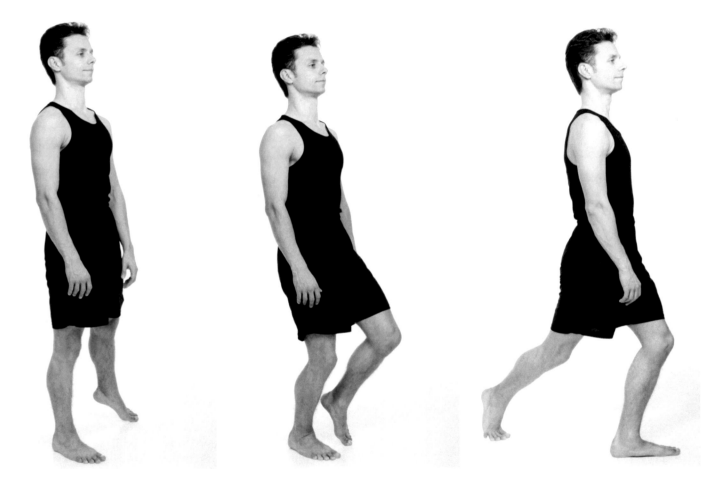

62. Shish Kabob

(Right over Right, Left over Left)

Purpose: To align the shoulder, rib and hip on each side for better balance, stability and efficiency of movement. Also, to make full weight transfers when taking a step (instead of weight being split).

Where Used: Everywhere.

Position: Standing.

1. Stand tall on your right leg. Imagine a skewer (stick) that runs from the top of your right shoulder blade down through the right side of your rib cage and pelvis, continuing down your right leg to your right heel. How vertical is your skewer?

2. Think of the left side of yourself as the meat on the skewer (i.e., your left shoulder, left side of your rib cage and pelvis, and your left leg). Keeping your skewer in place and vertical, begin to rotate the meat of your whole left side around it. Note that your spine is *not* the skewer—your spine is parallel to it. Then experiment with rotating just your shoulders and rib cage or just your pelvis around the skewer.

3. To feel the contrast, purposely allow your skewer to bend as you rotate the meat around it. Then return to rotating the meat around a straight skewer.

4. Repeat steps 1-3 standing on your left leg, using a left skewer.

5. Stand tall on your right leg, sensing your right skewer. Take a small side step to the left. Transfer weight to your left leg and establishing a straight left skewer (allow your right foot to brush to your left foot without weight). Then take a small side step to the right and re-establish your right skewer. Continue stepping side-brush, side-brush. Focus on moving from skewer to skewer without bending or breaking them.

6. Repeat step 5 stepping forward and back. Standing tall on your right leg, take a small step forward with your left foot (and establish the left skewer), then take a small step back with your

right foot (re-establishing the right skewer). After several times, switch to stepping the right foot forward (and left foot back). Pay attention to the various points along your skewers—shoulders, rib cage and pelvis. Do your skewers remain vertical or do they tilt as you take a step?

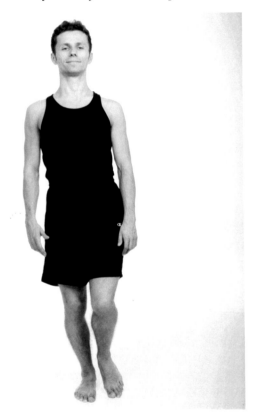 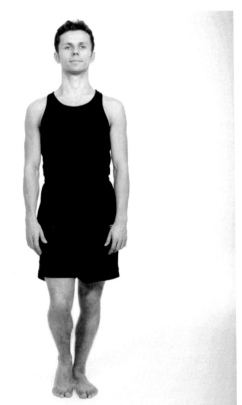

63. Johnnie Walker

(Walks in Smooth and Standard)

Purpose: To put the *Move Like a Champion®* principles to use in Smooth and Standard walks.

Where Used: All forward and back walks in Smooth and Standard.

Position: Standing.

Note: This exercise applies to forward and back walks in Waltz, Foxtrot, Viennese Waltz and Quickstep. In these dances the feet stay in contact with and skim the floor. In contrast, in Tango, the feet are slightly lifted off the floor and placed into position.

Forward Walks

1. Stand with feet together and weight on the right foot. Line up your blocks of weight (*Stack Up the Blocks*). Establish a neutral position of your pelvis (*Don't Get Tipsy*), rib cage (*Lace Up the Corset*), head and neck (*Knuckle Biter; Jewel of the Spine*). Allow your right foot to spread (*Grow a Shoe Size*).

2. With the ball of your left foot in contact with the floor, begin to swing your left leg forward from the hip joint without affecting the position of your pelvis (*Get a Leg Up; Turn on Your Headlights*). As your left foot moves forward, contact transitions from the ball of the foot to the whole foot. Allow the whole foot to lightly skim the floor as long as possible. At the same time, begin to release your right heel.

3. As your left knee begins to straighten, flex your left ankle in coordination (*Smooth Operator*). Your toes lift and your heel skims the floor (as in the heel lead part of *Feet with Attitude*).

4. Continue to skim your left heel on the floor, then stop at the mid-point of the stride. At this point, weight is equally divided between your left heel and the ball of your right foot. Your left knee is straight and your right knee is slightly flexed.

5. Continue to shift weight forward onto the left foot. Lower your left toes as you move your right foot forward, first with the toes, then the ball of the foot skimming the floor. At the completion of the step, your feet are together with weight fully transferred to your left foot.

6. Repeat steps 1-5 several times. Then switch legs (i.e., stand on your left foot and step forward with your right).

Back Walks

1. Do step 1 of the Forward Walks exercise.

2. Begin swinging your left leg backward from the hip joint without affecting the position of your pelvis (*Get a Leg Up; Turn on Your Headlights*). As your left foot moves back, first the ball of the foot is in contact with the floor, then the toes skim the floor. Then lower again onto the ball of the foot. As your left toes move past your right heel, begin to release your right toes from the floor.

   Don't forget to move your knees. On a left foot back step, your right knee moves forward in order to move your body back. Your left foot extends back one half of the distance of a full stride while lowering through both knees.

3. Your left foot arrives at the fullest extent of the stride after your knees finish lowering and your right knee straightens (your left knee remains slightly flexed). Your weight is equally divided between the ball of your left foot and the heel of your right foot.

4. Continue to shift your weight back onto the left foot. Do this by starting to move your right foot backward, first with the heel, and then with ball of the foot skimming the floor. As your right foot moves back, lower your left heel slowly and with control. When your weight is fully taken onto your left foot, your right foot is almost closed to your left foot without weight.

5. Repeat steps 1-4 several times. Then switch legs (i.e., stand on your left foot and step forward on your right).

Forward Walk in Waltz, Foxtrot, Viennese Waltz and Quickstep

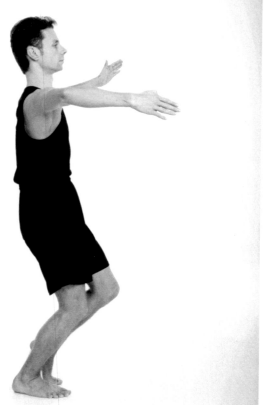

Preparation

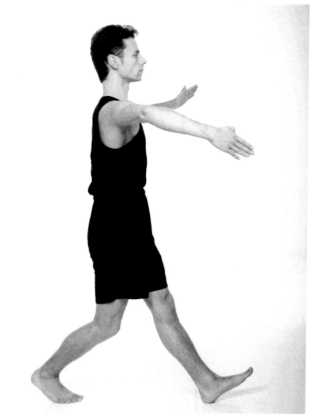

Mid-Point of Stride

Forward Walk in Tango

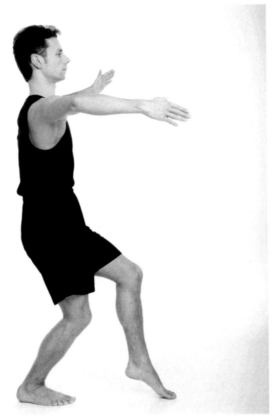

Preparation

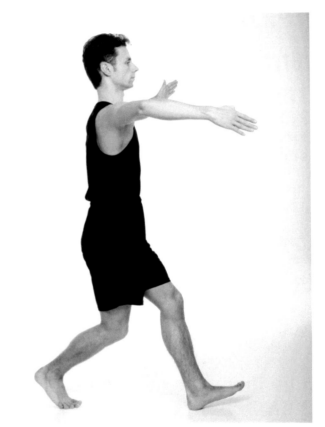

Mid-Point of Stride

64. Champion Latin and Rhythm Walks

(Walks in Rhythm and Latin)

Purpose: To put the *Move Like a Champion®* principles to use in Rhythm and Latin walks.

Where Used: Forward and back walks in Rhythm and Latin.

Position: Standing.

Forward Walks

1. Stand with your feet together and turned out. Transfer weight onto your right leg (have weight balanced on the front of your right heel and slightly toward the inside of the right foot). Bend your left knee (*Knee on a String*), allowing your left heel to come off the floor (toes stay connected to the floor). Observe that, at this moment, your pelvis is slightly tilted (*Rock the Boat* with the right side slightly higher) and turned to the right (*Bottle Brush*). The amount of rotation should match the turnout of the feet.

2. Start moving your weight forward through your standing right foot (*Guitar String Feet*). At the same time, begin to move your left leg forward, maintaining the bend in your knee. Without disturbing the alignment of your upper body, swing your left leg from the hip joint (*Get a Leg Up*) until the lower leg is perpendicular to the floor. Your left foot should be directly under your left knee (not left behind with the right foot). Your right knee remains straight yet soft.

3. Up to this point, the forward walk is the same in both the Latin and Rhythm dances. The difference happens now, when transferring weight. The dancer steps onto a straight leg in Latin and onto a bent leg in Rhythm.

International Latin: Swing your left shin (tibia) in front of your left knee, extending your left foot forward with the toes pointed and in contact with the floor. Then transfer your weight onto the left leg by rolling from the toes, through the ball, to the front of the left heel (*Guitar String Feet*; *Grow a Shoe Size*).

Simultaneously, peel your right heel off the floor, and then externally rotate your right leg (*Bottle Brush*). At the end of the walk, make sure your pelvis is level (*Don't Get Tipsy* and *Don't Rock the Boat*).

American Rhythm: Begin to transfer weight onto the ball (platform) of your left foot (*Barbie Feet*) with the left knee still bent and the right heel on the floor (also called a "delayed walk"). To fully transfer weight forward onto your left leg, lower your left heel and straighten your left knee. At the same time, allow your right heel to peel from the floor, and then externally rotate your right leg (*Bottle Brush*).

4.   Repeat steps 1-4, stepping forward on your right leg.

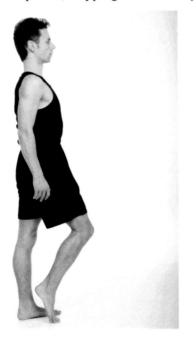 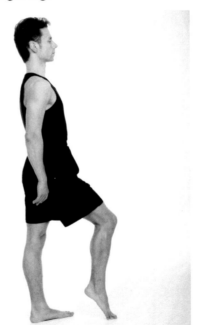 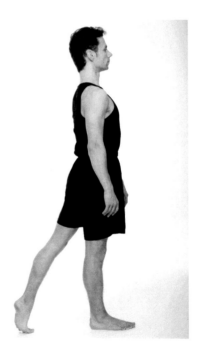

Back Walks

1. Stand with your feet together and turned out. Transfer weight onto your right leg (have weight balanced on the front of your right heel and slightly toward the inside of the right foot). Bend your left knee (*Knee on a String*), allowing your left heel to come off the floor (toes stay connected to the floor). Observe that, at this moment, your pelvis is slightly tilted (*Rock the Boat* with the right side slightly higher) and turned to the right (*Bottle Brush*). The amount of rotation should match the turnout of the feet.

2. Move your left leg backward from the hip joint, only as far as you are able to maintain a neutral pelvis (*Get a Leg Up*; *Don't get Tipsy*). Your left knee stays bent therefore your left foot goes farther back than your left knee. Keeping your pelvis level (*Don't Rock the Boat*), begin to shift your weight back along your right foot (*Guitar String Feet*), moving your whole self backward. Your right knee remains straight yet soft. Make sure not to drop the left side of your pelvis (*Don't Rock the Boat*).

3. Up to this point, the back walk is the same in both the Latin and Rhythm dances. The difference happens now, when transferring weight. The dancer steps onto a straight leg in Latin and onto a bent leg in Rhythm.

   International Latin: Straighten the left knee, extending the left foot farther back with toes pointed and touching the floor (make sure there is not too much turn out). Transfer weight onto your left foot, rolling from the toes, through the ball, to the front of the left heel. At this point, both legs should be straight with the right leg pointed in front.

   American Rhythm: Start transferring your weight onto the ball (platform) of your left foot (Barbie Feet) with the left knee bent (partial weight transfer). As you continue to transfer more weight onto your left leg, gradually lower your left heel while straightening your left knee. At the same time, bend your right knee and allow your right heel to lift from the floor (Smooth Operator). This causes your pelvis to tilt slightly—the right side will be slightly lower than the left side (Rock the Boat).

4. Repeat steps 1-4, stepping back with your right leg.

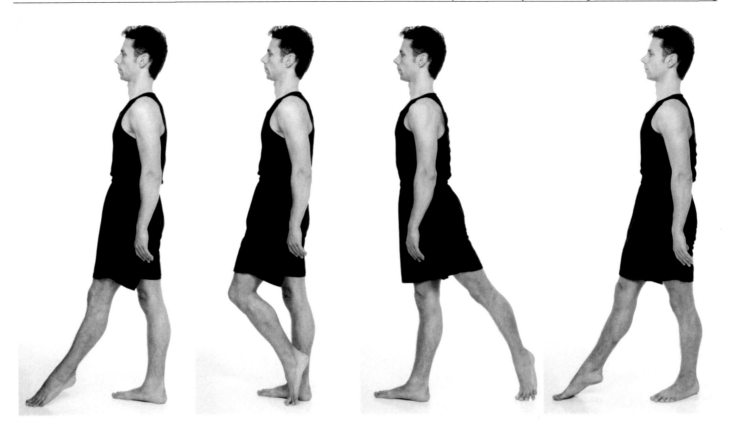

Top Pointers for Dynamic Alignment While Moving

1. Engage your abdominal muscles. This helps your torso to be lighter and better balanced so that your legs are able to move you more powerfully.

2. Focus on your standing (supporting) leg—this is a source of stability and power for your movement.

3. For the best balance and support, have weight in the frontmost part of your heel (not on your toes).

4. Take the time to do the preparatory movements *before* actually taking a step (*Going Without Going*).

5. When moving, make sure your pelvis stays in neutral (*Don't Get Tipsy* and *Turn on Your Headlights*) and your legs swing freely in the hip joints (*Get a Leg Up*).

6. In the Smooth and Standard dances, prepare *before* taking a step by lowering on your standing leg (*Put on Your PJs*).

7. Move your knees—powerful movement requires more mobility of the knees than most dancers realize (*Total Eclipse of the Toes; Smooth Operator*).

Study Guide

Joints (Use the following diagrams as study guides for the bones and joints.)

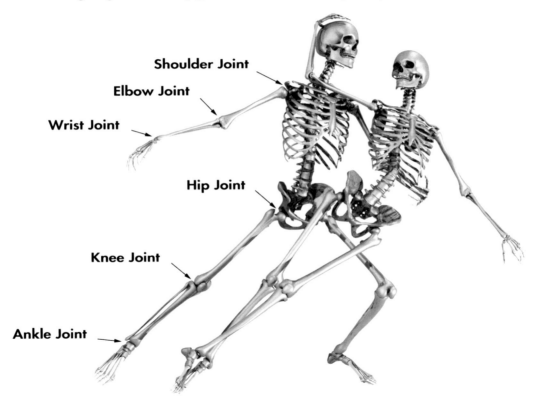

Shoulder Joint

Elbow Joint

Wrist Joint

Hip Joint

Knee Joint

Ankle Joint

Bones

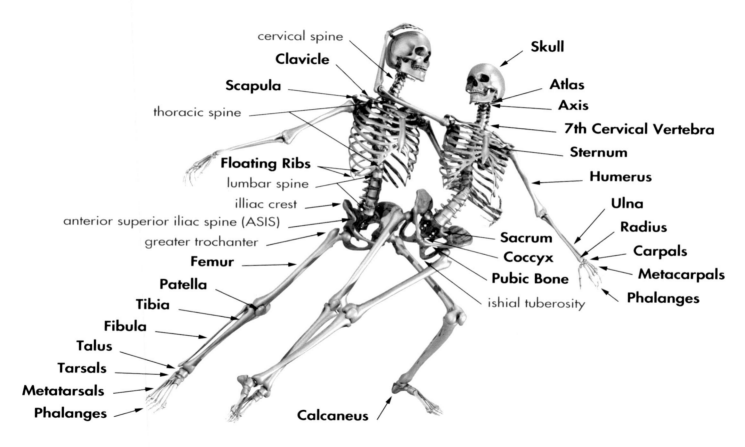

cervical spine
Clavicle
Scapula
thoracic spine

Floating Ribs
lumbar spine
illiac crest
anterior superior iliac spine (ASIS)
greater trochanter
Femur
Patella
Tibia
Fibula
Talus
Tarsals
Metatarsals
Phalanges

Calcaneus

Skull
Atlas
Axis
7th Cervical Vertebra
Sternum
Humerus
Ulna
Radius
Carpals
Metacarpals
Phalanges

Sacrum
Coccyx
Pubic Bone
ishial tuberosity

Test Yourself! (A circle at the start of an arrow indicates it is for a joint.)

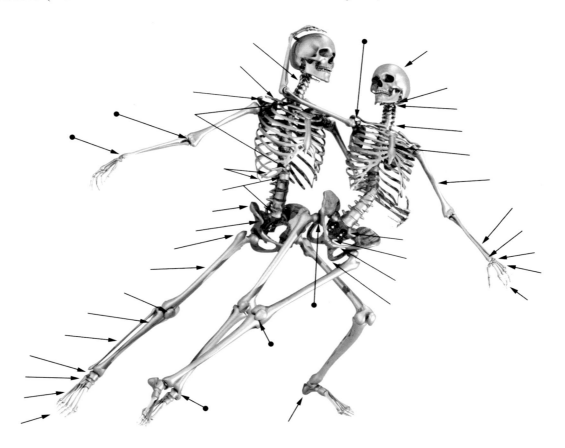

Notes

Notes

Notes

About the Authors

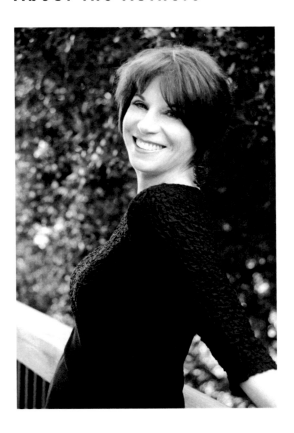

Diane Jarmolow

Diane Jarmolow is an innovator in the field of ballroom dancing. She founded the first ever vocational school for training ballroom dance teachers, the Ballroom Dance Teachers College. Her program *Ballroom Dance Teachers College-in-a-Box* is being presented in over 60 studios and universities throughout the United States, Canada, India, the Caribbean and Argentina. She is the author of *Teach Like a Pro®*, an encyclopedic book of information for dance teachers. She is the creator of the remarkable *Salesfree Sales* workshops designed to foster outstanding communication amongst teachers and students. Diane is a National Examiner with DVIDA®, and created their innovative system of professional certification. She authors the DVIDA® manuals, constantly improving the written language for ballroom dance. She also founded and operated San Francisco's enormously successful Metronome Ballroom. Diane's passion is helping people have the resources they need to become outstanding dance professionals and studio owners.

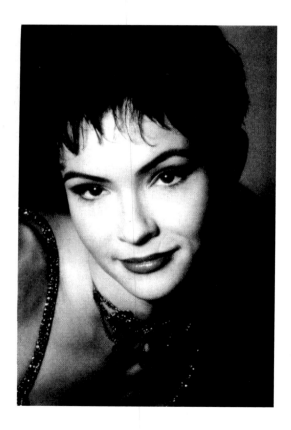

Kasia Kozak

Katarzyna Kozak, known as Kasia, is one of North America's most successful and beloved competitive ballroom dancers. Some of the highlights of her professional Latin dance competitive career with partners Donald Johnson, Andrew Phillips and Louis VanAmstel include:

•Blackpool Professional Latin Rising Star Champion

•Four-time U.S. National Professional Latin finalist

•Professional Latin Champion: Ohio Star Ball, Emerald Ball, Embassy Dancesport and Millenium Dancesport

Kasia's post-competitive career is every bit as exciting and dynamic as she continues to share her passion, enthusiasm and knowledge of dancing with dancers and teachers of all levels. Her unique brand *Kasia's High Heel Boot Camps* is widely recognized as achieving outstanding results for dancers seeking intensive dance training and invaluable insight into the mental side of competition preparation. Kasia has also created a variety of programs for studio managers to assist them in boosting student enthusiasm and participation, as well as ongoing teacher training. She is a mainstay teacher at Dance Mastery Dance Camps, and is featured in several popular dance training videos with her partner Donald Johnson.

Brandee Selck

A graduate of the Ballroom Dance Teachers College, Brandee Selck has been teaching ballroom dance for over 10 years. Brandee is also certified practitioner of the *Feldenkrais Method*®—movement education that utilizes our nervous system's ability to learn and change in order to improve movement and overall functioning. She brings her knowledge of *Feldenkrais*® to her dance teaching, as well as to developing educational materials and training curricula for the Ballroom Dance Teachers College, including *Ballroom Dance Teachers College-in-a-Box, Salesfree Sales* and *Teach Like a Pro*®. Brandee has also edited DVIDA® manuals and holds USISTD and DVIDA® certifications in American Smooth and a DVIDA® certification in American Rhythm.

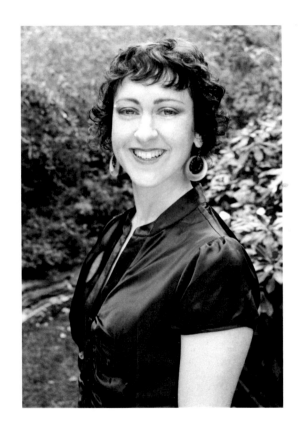

Resources

Training and Services by the Authors

Kasia Kozak offers Latin dance coaching and training intensives. **KasiaHighHeelsBootCamp.com**

Diane Jarmolow and the Ballroom Dance Teachers College offer teacher training, sales training, certification intensives and studio consulting. **TeachBallroomDancing.com**

Recommended Books

Teach Like a Pro®: The Ultimate Guide for Ballroom Dance Teachers by Diane Jarmolow with Brandee Selck, 2011.

Anatomy of Movement by Blandine Calais-Germain, 2007.

Dance, Mind and Body by Sandra Cerny Minton, 2003.

Dynamic Alignment Through Imagery (and other books) by Eric Franklin, 1996.

Luigis's Jazz Warm Up by Luigi, Lorraine Kriegel and Francis Roach, 1997.

Recommended Complimentary Practices

Bones for Life® ~ BonesForLife.com

Feldenkrais Method® ~ Feldenkrais.com

Iyengar Yoga ~ Iynaus.com

Nia Dance® ~ NiaNow.com

Z Health® Performance Solutions ~ ZHealth.net